BOND
WITH YOUR
BABY
BEFORE
BIRTH

How to Communicate With
Your Unborn Child

Kim O'Neill

Health Communications, Inc.
Deerfield Beach, Florida

www.hcibooks.com

Library of Congress Cataloging-in-Publication Data

O'Neill, Kim.

Bond with your baby before birth / Kim O'Neill.

    p. cm.

    Includes index.

    ISBN-13: 978-0-7573-0743-0 (trade paper)

    ISBN-10: 0-7573-0743-4 (trade paper)

    1. Motherhood.   2. Pregnancy.   3. Parent and infant.   4. Channeling

(Spiritualism)   I. Title.

HQ759.O626 2009

133.9—dc22

                                  2009002913

Publisher: Health Communications, Inc.

        3201 S.W. 15th Street

        Deerfield Beach, FL 33442–8190

Cover design by Justin Rotkowitz
Interior design and formatting by Lawna Patterson Oldfield

*With all my love I dedicate this book to
Flynn and Megan, the two intrepid souls who
chose me as a mother. The gift of their presence is a
greater happiness than I have ever known.
I also dedicate this book to my beautiful stepdaughter,
Jennifer, an incandescent being who is another
of my greatest earthly blessings.*

"She had seen their birth and the birth of her love for them as miraculous, but it was just as miraculous when they first smiled, first sat up, first babbled a sound that resembled, of course, mama. The tedious days were filled with miracles. When a baby first looks at you; when it gets excited about seeing a ray of light and like a dog pawing a gleam, tries to capture it with his hand; or when it laughs that deep, unselfconscious gurgle; or when it cries and you pick it up and it clings sobbing to you, saved from some terrible shadow moving across the room, or a loud clang in the street, or perhaps, already, a bad dream: then you are— happy is not the precise word—filled."

—*Marilyn French*
The Women's Room

CONTENTS

ACKNOWLEDGMENTS

Over the course of the last twenty-two years, I've conducted thousands of private channeling sessions for women from around the world who were in one of the three stages of creating the miracle of life: some were trying to conceive; others were already pregnant; and still others had already given birth to their little bundle of joy. I wish to acknowledge the clients who have allowed me to channel messages from their biological and adopted babies—both newborn and yet-be-born.

As clear as my psychic images were, my understanding about the entire process was always secondhand. It wasn't until my Mr. Wonderful finally arrived on the scene that I had the opportunity to gain firsthand knowledge about the magical, mystifying, hope-filled, and sometimes frustrating sequence of events that take place before, during, and after a baby is born. I was soon to discover that it is truly an experience like no other. Without my husband, Britt, this book would not have been possible.

I would like to thank my literary agent, Kirsten Manges, for her steadfast enthusiasm in the project and her guidance that helped shape and define the book that you now hold in your hands.

Without the support of Michele Matrisciani, my wonderful editor at HCI, this book could never have been born. I am eternally grateful to her.

Along the way, other earthly angels have supported and encouraged me, while still others have generously shared their stories: Jen Rogers, Brandie Walker, Tina Russell, Will LeBlanc, Julia Carroll, Bev Miller, Mike Beckman, Lisa Seales, Patti Calma, Anne Daley, Peggy Mendoza, Judy Hall, Michelle Bellamy, Melissa Hovey, Diane Porter, Melodie Joy, Sonya Dreikosen, Belin Jenkins, Rebecca Marina, Brenda Bostic, Kaia Klitzke, Susan Kirton, Remsey Nash, Dr. Vinaya Prabha V. Baligar, Winnie Baden, Tiffany Wignall, Nicola Kluge, Tara Nanayakkara, Carol Morris, Ali McDowell, Rebecca Kemble, Magdelena Wiebe, Shannon Jacobson, Ari McKinney, Aracelia "Tita" Valdes Gonzalez Vda de Rodriguez, Cheryle Rancourt, Kathy Hajovsky, Sharon St. Mary, Judy Fox, Certified Nurse Midwife Melanie Dossey, Dr. Elisa Medhus, Psychotherapist Carolyn H. Grace, and Dr. Geoffrey Schnider.

PREFACE

This book was written from my perspective as a professional channel with more than twenty-two years of experience in helping mothers-to-be learn how to bond with their unborn babies.

Think of me as your very own spiritual coach. As one mother to another, I'll support you in building the all-important bond between you and your child, and facilitate your understanding of his needs, challenges, likes, and dislikes . . . and even his special destiny. Accessing this vital information will also help you discover the specific reasons why your baby deliberately chose you as a mother, which can serve to alleviate fears and concerns you may have about the kind of mother you'll be.

The book you now hold in your hands can help you open a dialogue with the incredible soul who is destined to be your child. In Chapter Five, you'll find my simple step-by-step technique that will allow you to develop a two-way line of communication with your unborn baby. In Chapter Six, I provide you with a comprehensive list of questions that you can pose to your unborn baby that can help jumpstart the back-and-forth communication.

While navigating your spiritual path, you'll have the privilege of being exposed to many different schools of thought. As you continue to explore all of the unique philosophies and messages conveyed in books, films, plays, and art—and espoused through professionals in the spiritual sciences—I believe that it's important to embrace what feels right to you.

The seeds that you plant today in your spiritual garden will yield a lifetime of blooms, as long as you remain open and curious about the world around you. Change is as inevitable as the passing of seasons. You have within you the ability to cultivate your spiritual garden so that it flourishes fuller and brighter with each new season of your life. To be receptive to new thoughts and ideas throughout one's existence on the earthly plane is what markedly defines an enlightened human being.

What I am presenting within these pages are my truths. Thank you for allowing me to share them with you.

ONE

HOW BONDING BEGINS

Chapter Profile: The spirit of your baby is nearby, eager to begin his new life with you. When you're pregnant, your psychic ability expands as quickly as your waistline! Chapter One introduces you to the process of speaking with the spirit of your future child. My fervent hope is that this book will allow you to become more sensitive to the presence of your unborn baby as he or she hovers around you. Think of me as a personal coach who can help you embark on a spiritual adventure unlike any you've ever known . . . on the path that leads directly toward the magical experience of bonding with the soul of your unborn baby.

When does the bonding process begin? There are probably as many opinions about that as there are . . . people!

Belin's Story

When I have tuned into my womb, and even deeper into the soul of my baby, I have felt a connection that transcends time and mind. It's a heart connection and a knowing. You just have to trust in that communication. The more practice you have communicating with your little baby in utero, the better able you will be able to connect when that little soul is born. When does the connection start? It starts when we allow it. I discovered that you don't even have to be pregnant to feel it.

My opinion resonates from a *metaphysical* viewpoint. Based upon my life's work as a channel and through my own experience giving birth, I believe that bonding begins when a soul first starts to hover around its chosen birth mother, even if she remains unaware of its presence, isn't pregnant yet—or has even yet to meet a Mr. Wonderful.

Dr. Schnider, a father and grandfather who has delivered more than seven thousand babies in his twenty-eight-year career as an obstetrician, has formed an opinion about mother/baby bonding stemming from a *scientific* viewpoint. "I think women start bonding fairly early," he told me. "Once she sees the baby on ultrasound, when she sees the actual heartbeat, it makes a much bigger impact than just 'feeling.' And then another big step is when she feels movement . . . they're bonded."

Your baby will be your greatest blessing. My fervent hope is that this book will allow you to become more sensitive to the presence of your unborn baby. The key to building a constructive relationship is to maintain faith that your baby is eager to connect, and to accept the fact that you already possess all of the skills necessary to build the two-way communication. By practicing the technique in the fifth chapter, you'll hone your ability to better hear the vital messages your unborn baby has been trying to convey—possibly even before you conceived. The bonding will become increasingly tangible—and therefore, more exciting!

I have worked as a psychic for over twenty-two years, delivering angelic messages for clients in private channeling sessions. I've channeled for people from all over the world and in very different walks of life. Through the years, clients have asked about their careers, life's work, soul mates, health, financial abundance, family members, as well as many other topics. My life's purpose is to help people gain valuable insight into who they are; what they are supposed to be doing with their lives; the specific, pragmatic steps they can take to reach their full potential; and how they can create the empowerment necessary to build a lovely quality of life.

How did I begin to communicate with the souls of unborn babies? It all began one miraculous day shortly after I became a professional psychic. I was conducting a private channeling session for a pregnant client, and she was asking her angels for information about her prenatal health. As I listened to the telepathic messages coming from her angels in answer to her question, I was surprised to hear another voice say, "Hi, Mommy!" I was mystified. I asked if the voice was one of her angels, and I heard the message, "No, I am the spirit of her daughter." I repeated this surprising information to my client. She asked if the message was coming from the soul who was going to actually become her child. "Yes!" responded the spirit. "And I can't wait to be born!"

I quickly realized that the process of communicating with the souls of unborn babies is *exactly* the same as speaking with guardian angels, and simple to learn—with just a little practice. Throughout the years, I made another startling discovery: after conception, a woman's natural intuitiveness dramatically strengthens and deepens, allowing her to become far more psychically receptive to what is going on around her during her pregnancy.

In this book, I'm sharing information revealed in private channeling sessions conducted with expectant mothers from all over the world—true-life stories about parents who began the bonding process before their babies were conceived, or after they were in utero—as well as what I experienced throughout my own two pregnancies.

I have to admit that *my* story is a little unusual. Instead of meeting my husband, Britt, in a bookstore, through a friend, or even online, I met him for the first time when he came into my office asking me to channel the spirit of his recently deceased wife! Not exactly the romantic vision that I had always dreamed of. Plus, I was already forty years old at the time. In spite of—or, maybe *because* of—what brought us together, love blossomed and we were married three months later. Britt had a grown daughter and wanted more children, and I was keen to finally start a family. Although I did not realize it at the time, the spirit of my unborn son was already hovering around me . . . even before I conceived!

This is the true story of the very first time I communicated with my own unborn child:

I arrived at the doctor's office for my annual pap smear, was shown to an exam room, donned a blue paper gown, and sat waiting for my doctor. Dr. Schnider, my OB/GYN, entered the room and greeted me with a warm smile, as always. He apologized for keeping me waiting—explaining that he had delivered a baby that morning so he was running a little behind schedule. As he reviewed my chart, he asked how I was feeling and I told him that I had never felt better. Then it was time for the internal.

When he finished, I sat up on the exam table and told him that since my last visit, I had finally met my Mr. Wonderful and had gotten married. The doctor offered hearty congratulations. Then I told him that we were going to try to get pregnant. My dreams were all coming true, I giggled. Dr. Schnider's expression seemed to cloud for a brief moment. He asked me to meet him in his office once I had dressed. With a nod, he left the room.

I dressed and walked into the hallway where Janet, the nurse, was waiting for me. Janet told me that the doctor had to take an emergency call, so he would be a few minutes. She ushered me into a tiny waiting room directly outside his private office. Photographs of the babies Dr. Schnider had delivered lined all of the walls. In some, he was still in his scrubs, cheerfully holding infants that had just been born. I was immediately entranced by that wall of babies. My children would have their picture on that wall, too, I decided happily. I fantasized about what my children would be like in temperament and appearance, excited about the future of my personal life and all of its endless possibilities.

Lost in this train of blissful thought, I was startled when Janet touched my arm to get my attention. She led me to the doctor's private office and gestured for me to take a seat. He would be there momentarily, she said, leaving me alone in the room. Why was I there? Tapping my foot with impatience, I began to look around. Some large photos on his credenza were of smiling teenagers, and I guessed that they were his children. I wasn't surprised to see how good looking all of them were.

Dr. Schnider rushed into the office, this time with more apologies about keeping me waiting. He disclosed that one of his other patients was laboring in the Women's Hospital across the street and he was preparing to help her deliver that evening. The doctor explained that he had been rushing back and forth between the hospital and his office all morning. I felt guilty that I had been so impatient.

"I want to share something with you," he said softly, opening a drawer of his credenza. He pulled out what appeared to be several graphs and placed them on the desk between us. I just stared dumbly, having no idea what he was trying to communicate. His expression was so somber that my heart started to pound.

Suddenly, I didn't want to see them. I just sat motionless. He kindly waited for a few moments and then picked them up himself. He sat forward in his chair so he could hold them up for me to see. They were charts depicting a woman's fertility levels at age twenty. Then I understood. The doctor intended to discuss my biological clock.

The chart pointed out that at the ripe old age of thirty-five a woman's fertility starts to sink like a lead balloon. I was already over forty. I looked at the chances of fertility for someone my age . . . and the line of fertility plummeted to ground zero. My heart sank.

But how could that be, I wondered? I had never tried to get pregnant before, but I just assumed that I still had plenty of eggs left. Dr. Schnider gently pointed out that because I had delayed pregnancy, it might be more difficult for me to conceive, that there was an increased possibility of genetic abnormalities, and that I had a higher risk of miscarriage. He told me that as his patient, he wanted me to be as informed as possible.

Instead of being grateful for his honesty, I felt as if I had been hit in the solar plexus. I had never considered *any* of these realities! The doctor, observing my distress, reassured me that, if necessary, there were fertility options open to me. But my mind was spinning and I was no longer listening to him.

In the past, my priority had been *preventing* pregnancy because I hadn't met Mr. Wonderful. Now that he had finally come into my life, it appeared as though my dreams of a family might be cruelly over before they could even take shape.

An immense wave of sadness and loss washed over me. A big lump began to form in my throat as my eyes welled up with tears. I dug in my purse for a handful of tissues. I told Dr. Schnider that I needed to think, and without another word, I fled past the nurse's desk and into the reception area, past all the pregnant patients waiting for their prenatal appointments, and out into the hallway.

I couldn't make it to the public bathroom down the corridor. I burst into a flood of tears, standing right there in the middle of the hallway. I had been completely unprepared for the dreadful sense of loss and the "but why me?" disbelief that I might not be able to have the opportunity to have a child. I had always taken it for granted as my female prerogative; that someday, whenever I was ready, I would get pregnant and have a baby. It truly never occurred to me that my opportunity could expire prematurely before menopause. Like a lot of other women over thirty-five, I had chosen to relegate my fertility to the back of a figurative closet like a beautiful hat that didn't quite fit me yet, while telling myself that it would always be there when I needed it.

What was I going to *do*? Should I get a second opinion . . . in spite of the fact that Dr. Schnider was the chief of staff of Texas Woman's Hospital and had a reputation as *the* pre-eminent OB/GYN in Houston? I knew intuitively that he was the very best doctor for me; after all, my angels had directed me to him. Would I have to endure years of painful, expensive fertility treatments? Where would we get the money? What if they didn't work?

Still standing in the hallway, now propped up against the wall, I started to sob even harder. Maybe I shouldn't have waited until I met Mr. Wonderful. Had I made a huge mistake? I thought of the men I had dated over the dismal years when I was single—and clearly, none of them had ever been my idea of a good candidate for the father of my children. I had been married before, but my ex-husband made no secret of the fact that he had as much interest in having a child with me as he did climbing Mt. Everest without a canister of oxygen. Now that I did have a heart, mind, body, and soul relationship, my age was the saboteur. The tears were still streaming when I was soundly bumped from behind by a little boy who was quickly and quietly chastised by his mother, and I realized that I had to get out of the busy hallway.

I scurried to the ladies room, found an empty stall, squeezed inside, and sat on the toilet with my purse in my lap. I grabbed some tissue and loudly blew my nose. I morosely thought of my new husband. I was going to dash all of Britt's dreams about having a child with me. Maybe he should find a younger woman? Why hadn't he come into my life sooner? Why couldn't I have what so many other women have? Why was my personal life always so impossibly difficult? Why . . .

"Stop! Kim! You need to listen! You will have a child!" My guardian angel, John, was shouting telepathically; I could hear his words clearly inside my head.

"How is that possible?" I wailed aloud, not caring who could hear me. "Dr. Schnider said—"

"There are other factors involved!" my angel insisted. *"Your destiny was to have your children later in life! We've talked about that!"*

"But the doctor is an experienced fertility expert, and maybe—"

"Haven't we told you that first . . . you were destined to meet your Mr. Wonderful . . . and then you were going to start your family?"

"Yes," I sniffed.

"And before you met Britt, how many times did you tell us that you didn't really believe you would ever meet a romantic soul mate?"

"A lot," I conceded.

"And the soul mate came, and now you are happily married. Didn't that happen as we told you it would?"

"Yes, that's true," I whined. "But now—"

"Although what you thought was impossible has already come to pass,

you now doubt that the next part of your destiny will materialize. How can someone who channels as a life's work have such an issue with faith?"

"I don't know," I cried, shaking my head. "I'm so depressed."

"Why don't I introduce the new spirit hovering around you?"

"All right," I replied, without enthusiasm, feeling very sorry for myself. "I suppose I need all the angelic help I can get right now."

"This spirit is planning on getting help from you."

"Huh? How could I help a spirit?"

"Hi, Mom!" said a childlike, disembodied voice.

"Who is *that?*" I asked.

"I can't wait to be your son!" answered the voice.

"John . . . who is that speaking to me?"

"Your future offspring," the angel told me.

"You mean, my *baby?*"

"Hi, Mom, I'm right here!"

"Oh, my God . . . then I can really have children?"

"Isn't that what we've always told you?" chided John.

"You're going to be a little boy?" I asked the spirit, now sobbing again.

"Yes—your little boy!" said the childlike voice. *"I'm coming first!"*

"Does that mean I'm going to have a second child?"

"My sister is coming next . . . but I get to come first!"

"Really?" I asked. "I'm going to have a son . . . *and* a daughter?"

"All kinds of rapturous things are continually happening behind the scenes that human beings are unaware of," John reminded me.

"This is the best news I've ever had! Will I have any problems getting pregnant?"

"None at all," John confirmed. *"But you have to be patient! Remember, each soul decides when he or she will be born. That is not your decision. However, you must do your part."*

"Can I talk to my baby any time I want?"

"Yes," said John. *"All souls hover around their chosen birth mother to begin the bonding process before birth."*

"This spirit chose me as a mom?" I asked, incredulous. "Why did he pick *me*?"

"Because you'll love me and support me and help me get into my life's work," said my unborn child. *"And because I need your help with a big issue . . . patience. I'm not as patient as you are!"*

My eyes widened. I heard John chuckle.

"May God help you both," remarked the angel, clearly amused.

"I need to call Britt right away!" I said, my hands shaking as I fumbled inside my purse for the cell phone. My husband answered on the second ring.

"Sweetie!" I cried. "It's me! Guess *what*?"

"Are you crying?" asked Britt.

"Don't worry!" I sniffed. "Everything is going to be okay!"

"What did the doctor say?"

"Dr. Schnider warned me that we have some major hurdles to overcome."

Silence.

"Guess who's here with me?"

"Are you still in the doctor's office?" he inquired worriedly.

"No, I'm in the toilet."

Silence.

"My angel John is here! And I just talked to our *baby*! He's going to be a boy! And he told me that I'm going to help him develop patience! Isn't that *funny*?"

Silence.

"I'll be there as soon as I can! We've got important work to do! I love you!" Without waiting for his response, I closed my cell phone, wiped the last of my tears, got up and strode out of the bathroom, with John and the spirit of my little boy in close pursuit. I was in a hurry. Britt and I were going to make a baby!

Fast forward to the time I was in my eighth month of pregnancy. It was then that I realized that I wouldn't know what to do once the baby arrived. Waves of fear gripped me. Although I was very nurturing and mature, I wasn't exactly Suzy Homemaker. I had nightmarish images of my child as an adult sitting in a therapist's office, sobbing, "Do you know what it was like to grow up as the child of a professional *psychic* . . . who never cooked? All I ate was carry-out! My life is ruined!"

It's amusing to me now, but I was truly concerned that I wouldn't be able to *do* it. I had never even *held* a baby before. Thank God I already had years of experience channeling for other pregnant women. So, I simply put my expertise to work and began to speak with *my* unborn baby. When he told me that he wanted to come to me more than anything else in the world, it really helped quell some of my worst fears. The more the baby reassured me throughout the pregnancy—about his health, my health, and the future—the better I felt.

When conducting private channeling sessions for women who

were trying to conceive, or for women who were already expecting, there were always many questions that the mother-to-be was keen to have answered by her angels, or the unborn baby himself: Will my pregnancy be okay? Will the baby be healthy? Will I be healthy? What will I experience during labor and delivery? What about the baby's name? What color should I paint the nursery? Should I breast-feed or give him formula? Is there anything in the house that will scare him . . . like the dog? How can I help him with his issues? What will my child choose as his profession when he grows up?

As an expectant mother, wouldn't you *love* to know the answers to these questions and countless others . . . *before* your little one arrives? You *can*, by developing a better understanding of how and when spiritual beings—such as your unborn child and guardian angels—communicate with you.

Every time I conduct a seminar or workshop, someone always raises their hand and declares, "You're going to think I'm crazy, but . . .", and then they relay an amazing story about how they *knew* they had a supernatural encounter with their unborn child, one of their guardian angels, or even a deceased friend or family member. The audience listens with rapt attention until that individual once again takes her seat; then, suddenly, a flurry of hands shoot up as other people eagerly wish to share their own personal metaphysical experiences.

What I've learned as a professional psychic is that we all have spiritual beings hovering around us—whether we realize it or not. Do you know there is a very thin veil between the earthly plane, where human beings reside, and the heavenly plane that is home to spiritual beings? This means that we can freely communicate with beings that live in heaven, and *they* can convey messages to us, which they do on a regular basis. These messages can have a profound effect on the entire quality of your life. Spiritual beings are primarily made up of three distinct groups: the soul of your unborn baby, guardian angels, and the departed.

THE SOUL OF YOUR UNBORN BABY

The first group consists of your unborn babies who are happily and consistently present once they have chosen you as a mother.

GUARDIAN ANGELS

The second group of spiritual beings is comprised of the guardian angels who serve, protect, and guide you.

THE DEPARTED

The third group includes loved ones who have passed away, including departed friends, family members—and, yes, even your pets!

Consider the probability that *right now*, you have any number of spiritual beings attempting to communicate with you. This communication between human beings and spiritual beings is commonly referred to as *channeling*. And just because you may remain unaware of their presence does not mean they are not there.

While I'm conducting a private session, I'll often "see" a poignant picture in my mind's eye of a client's deceased loved one holding an unborn child on their knee, or playing with the baby, sometimes even long before conception occurs. Because we all continue to incarnate with one another, we enjoy interacting with those with whom we share long-standing relationships—whether we exist in heaven or on earth.

While your deceased loved ones may visit for short periods at a time, both your unborn baby and your guardian angels communicate with you around the clock. They provide information typically through the process of telepathy, which means the spiritual messages simply "pop" into your head—as if you were talking to yourself. Your unborn baby and angels can also communicate with you *on the fly* while you are going about your daily routine, and if you have a jam-packed schedule racing from one task or obligation to another, you might get some of their messages confused with your own thoughts.

That is the reason I strongly recommend that you consider making the time to sit down and practice your ability to communicate with them. If you set aside no more than half an hour a week to find a quiet place and open a dialogue with your baby-to-be and guardian angels, you will be astonished at how quickly your channeling skills can blossom. Conducting my fun, easy, and simple practicing techniques will be your secret to success. Think of it as meditating. It is the most productive method by which you can receive intuitive messages because you are not distracted by outside stimuli.

Were you aware that throughout your life, the majority of your gut instincts and some of your creative ideas come from the communication you receive from your angels? Of course, you also receive intuitive information from your unborn baby while he hovers around you between the time he has chosen you as a mother and the time he is born. This is why I encourage you to begin focusing on the two-way communication without delay—even if you aren't pregnant yet! In fact, your baby may choose you as a mother *years* before you actually conceive. Imagine how remarkable it will feel the very first time your baby is placed in your arms—and the joyful familiarity that is likely to pass between you!

Are you aware that you're already an accomplished channel? This is because your guardian angels have been communicating with you telepathically since you were born. They speak with you at night when you're asleep in the form of dreams, as well as while you are awake and going about your daily routine.

Angelic messages are conveyed to you in a constant stream of information. That's why it seems like you are talking to yourself *all the time*. What you're really doing is speaking with your guardian angels. So it stands to reason that you are fully capable of receiving channeled messages from your unborn baby. It's exactly the same process.

In addition, as you practice, the relationship between you, your unborn baby, and your guardian angels may become increasingly tangible. Some people—like me—yearn to see and *hear* spiritual beings. I have had a number of clients who have told me that after they spent a brief period of time talking with their unborn baby and guardian angels, they could actually hear their *voices*. Others have experienced spiritual beings materializing right in front of them! But please don't worry if you're an individual who might be frightened by that. Your unborn baby and guardian angels typically wait to tangibly materialize until you ask them.

Another time in which you are very receptive to spiritual visitations is while you sleep. Your unborn child and angels consider you much more open to receiving their communication at that time because you are a captive audience. Your brain doesn't interrupt the flow of your channeling by repeatedly announcing, "This is impossible—it can't be happening!" Many of your dreams convey special messages. At times, when you are sleeping, your unborn child, your angels, and departed loved ones may appear visually, in your mind's eye, speaking directly to you to build and maintain a close spiritual and emotional bond. After one of their visits, whether you have total recall of the dream or not, you are likely to wake up feeling very refreshed, peaceful, and rested, ready to start the day with a more positive and optimistic outlook—as if you've just returned from a three-week vacation!

You might be wondering how communicating with spiritual beings, like your unborn baby or guardian angels, might support—or contradict—your religious beliefs. A number of religions promote the existence of heaven—where your unborn baby now exists—and a number of religions subscribe to the existence of guardian angels.

I believe that angels are messengers from God, sent to guide our spiritual evolution and help direct us toward the purpose in which we can best help our fellow man. I also believe that souls never "die," but instead continue to live, whether on earth or in heaven.

Whichever religion you follow, have faith that you'll *know* what feels right to you. The philosophies you choose to embrace in regard to religion or spirituality are a very personal choice. What feels right to you may conflict with what feels right to your parents, siblings, friends, fellow parishioners, or even spouse. Open yourself to exploring new and different philosophies. Rest assured that it's very unlikely that you'd consider any philosophy that doesn't dovetail or coincide with your inborn sensibilities, ethics, or sense of honor.

I'm fascinated by the seismic shift of consciousness that is sweeping the nation. America has widened its horizons to embrace a passionate focus on metaphysical topics such as angels, psychic ability, channeling, and holistic healing. A recent Gallup News Service poll reported that half of all Americans believe in extrasensory perception, and psychic, or spiritual, healing. More than 20 million Americans believe they have seen a ghost, and according to a *Life Magazine* article about angels, "69 percent of Americans believe they exist."

As you continue on your special journey, consider the fact that you have the opportunity of choosing a philosophy that is strictly religious, which is the practice of an organized faith; or entirely spiritual, which is the practice of pursuing beliefs outside of religious doctrine; or a combination of the two—as long as they feel right to you.

Even the most conservative people you know who dismiss anything related to metaphysics have guardian angels and unborn babies hovering around them who are attempting to convey vitally important messages to help them build a better quality of life. Regardless of whether someone chooses to believe in their presence, spiritual beings remain present—and accounted for!

I believe that children are the best channels on the earthly plane because they do not discount or dismiss what they hear from spirits. That is the reason so many departed loved ones and unborn babies choose to interact with children *before* communicating with the adults in the family—as illustrated in the true-life stories throughout this book. Interestingly, it is often the young children who approach Mom or Dad to share the news about a new baby coming, sometimes even before Mom conceives. It's also been my professional (and personal) experience that children can often intuit everything that's going on in the household, regardless of how successfully you believe that they're being shielded from certain realities, such as marital discord or pesky financial challenges.

Your unborn babies are eager to connect with their siblings who are living on the earthly plane. Sometimes they will visit their big brothers or sisters in dreams, or they might appear, tangibly, to play with them. They may even be accompanied by departed loved ones.

Diane's Story

When my granddaughter, Katie, was just a little over two years old, her mother overheard her talking excitedly to her teddy bear. "Baby's coming! Baby's coming!"

The next time Katie visited my house, I asked her, "Katie, is a baby coming?" "Yes . . . a baby brother," she informed me. "Are you excited?" I inquired. "Yes!" she squealed, wide-eyed. My daughter was pregnant three months later and delivered a healthy baby boy.

You can foster your child's growing awareness and curiosity in the spiritual beings that surround him—including his guardian angels, your family's departed loved ones, and his unborn sibling(s)—simply by acknowledging the process. Then continually encourage your children to talk about what they have "heard" or "sensed" from spirit. Consider a spiritual play date each week for you and your already-born child to sit together and engage unborn children, loved ones in spirit, and his angels in a conversation. You will be amazed at the wealth of information that is channeled through your little ones!

Besides supporting the connection with their angels and loved ones who are no longer on the earthly plane, you'll be proactively cultivating a growing connection between your already-born earthly children and unborn babies that will help them feel more of a bond once the birth takes place. For example, if you explain to your children that the new brother or sister has come all the way from heaven to play with them, then sibling rivalry, regressive behavior, and fighting for Mom's attention might be partially circumvented . . . which will be yet another blessing for you.

Michelle's Story

When I was pregnant the first time, I knew the day I conceived. There was something magic in the air. It was like electricity, energy. Jason and I were not actively trying to have a baby, although we had just bought a house together and had eloped. We were leaving to go on our Hawaiian honeymoon a few weeks later, and I felt pregnant.

I knew the baby was a girl and that we would call her Madison. I talked to her all the time and called her by name. We had an ultrasound that confirmed that I was right, it was a girl. Madison is now nine years old. She remembers a time before she was born and has told me about it. She also remembers being inside of me and not wanting to come out at the hospital. She was finally born via c-section.

Madison had stronger communications with my youngest daughter, Alyssa, in utero than I did. She chose her name and told me they knew each other before they were born; but Madison told her she needed to go first, because she knew more than her.

As a Natural Childbirth Educator in the Hypnobabies Method, I have done work with women who are pregnant or trying to get pregnant, and when I've had communications with their babies, it is always so special to me.

If there is no one currently in your life who believes that it's possible to communicate or develop a relationship with your unborn baby, I respectfully submit to you that it isn't necessary to obtain anyone else's permission, approval, or endorsement to believe in whatever philosophies or sensibilities you choose. Rest assured that there will be at least one family member, friend, coworker, or even your doctor who thinks you're nutty when you tell them that you think it's possible to communicate with your unborn baby; but it won't be the first time, I'm sure, that they think you're a little "around the bend." Nor will it be the last! No matter *what* topic you introduce to another person, there is likely to be a difference of outlook and opinion.

There are as many differences of opinions as there are topics to discuss. For example, are there specific topics you know not to mention during family gatherings, or arguing is sure to erupt—or at least a lot of raving and ranting? That's one of the reasons family reunions or holiday gatherings can be, at times, a little stressful. My mom is still very angry with my alcoholic, abusive dad, although it's been more than thirty years since they got a divorce. The mere mention of his name is sure to make sparks fly. My brother Michael is very sensitive to a certain newsworthy person who he considered disloyal to the United States during the Vietnam War—although Michael was just a small child at the time of that conflict. Just mention this person's name and my brother starts to rave. For my part, because of my prior lifetime during the Holocaust, I jump into the fray the moment I hear someone criticized because of their race, religion, or gender. If someone was to disparage Indiana Jones (or Harrison Ford), my eight-year-old son would give them a piece of his mind! Bring up the U.S. tax system, and my normally mild-mannered husband flies into a tizzy . . . and everybody wishes that he had an off switch! For her part, my stepdaughter Jennifer, an attorney, wants to prevail over the proponents of capital punishment and will speak passionately about that topic.

We all have our interests, beliefs, passions, opinions, and philosophies. Enlightened individuals can speak their truths and allow others to speak theirs—regardless of whether they hold the same beliefs. However, there are times when someone will choose to argue with you over a specific belief that you embrace in an effort to prove you wrong or an attempt to manipulate you into believing as they do. Some people just love to argue and will always give the impression that they have to be "right," and that nobody else knows more than they do.

Whenever I meet someone who obviously embraces a very different truth, I will sometimes choose to remain quiet—just to maintain my inner peace and avoid a nonsensical conflict. We are all repeatedly faced with this question: do we choose to avoid an argument or discussion by remaining quiet about what we believe, or do we speak up and calmly state our opinions even if others believe differently than we do? In any case, how much do we really need the permission, endorsement, or acknowledgement of others to embrace the beliefs that feel good to us?

If you're currently expecting a baby, *this is the moment* to begin connecting with the soul of the little being who will soon join your family. If you're trying to get pregnant—or you're in the adoption process—you may already have one or more unborn babies hovering around you. Your baby is already trying to convey messages to you. Have you been receiving them? Don't wait until the baby is born. Begin the precious bonding process . . . right now!

—

TWO

DISCOVERING THE JOURNEY OF YOUR BABY'S SOUL

Chapter Profile: You'll be one step further to communicating with your unborn baby by learning about reincarnation—which explains *how* and *where* your baby is living . . . right now!

Do you wonder where the soul of your unborn baby is living right now? Or how he is getting the nurturing he needs without you? If he does not have a physical body, how does he *exist*? Can he really see and hear you? Do you wonder when his soul will enter the tiny physical body that is growing inside of you?

REINCARNATION AND YOUR BABY

The process of a soul traveling from heaven to earth, and from earth to heaven, is called reincarnation. The soul, or spirit, of your baby is making this extraordinary journey for the purpose of improving himself and evolving spiritually—which he will accomplish only with your help. Your unborn baby is journeying from heaven to earth, in good part, to be with *you*.

You are going to provide the means by which another soul, who has chosen you as a parent, will return to the earthly plane to fulfill a destiny that he has already mapped out. Your new awareness of the challenging transition process will allow you to offer him the support, guidance, and encouragement that he will so desperately need from you as his parent to help him reach his full potential and create a life that will make his heart and soul sing. At the same time, you have a responsibility to build a life that you can love. I believe that as mothers, our babies have a way of fulfilling us like nothing else!

Let's begin our discussion of reincarnation by describing the two very different places that your baby's soul can exist: heaven and earth. Your unborn baby's soul remains fully alive—for all eternity—regardless of whether he lives in heaven or on earth. However, heaven is the center of where the reincarnation process takes shape.

In my experience as a channel, I have spoken with many guardian angels and the spirits of departed human beings. They have told me that heaven is an actual *place*, and it is where your baby lives right now as a spiritual being along with God, his angels, and all of your departed loved ones. It is the home to all noncorporeal beings in between their earthly lifetimes. Therefore, all beings reside in one of two places: in heaven as a spirit, or on earth as a human being.

When your baby resides in heaven—like now, before he is

born—he does not have a physical body. He is a spirit. Your baby's spirit, or soul, looks like a ball or beam of light.

Throughout the years, I've had many clients ask what heaven is like. They want to know what I've learned as a channel, speaking with spiritual beings every day.

First of all, I've been told by guardian angels that in heaven it is effortless to manifest what you most desire. If you wish to live in an environment that resembles the seashore, or the mountains, you will find yourself there simply by focusing on that desire. If you wish to form relationships with a soul mate, friends, or family—who are also spirits living in heaven—you can draw them to you simply by focusing on that desire. If you wish to perform a certain kind of work—such as being a guardian angel—you may focus on that desire to turn it into a reality.

Anything you wish is at your immediate disposal—except for one thing. In heaven, you cannot work through any issues or develop greater enlightenment because there is no adversity there. In heaven, all souls act at the highest level of the enlightenment they already have, meaning that they are as unfailingly generous, supportive, encouraging, and loving with one another as they are capable of being at that time. As wonderful as this is, at the same time, it creates an interesting dilemma. Without adversity, a soul cannot evolve. So, from time to time, souls who wish to evolve plan to make the journey to the earthly plane—where there is plenty of adversity to help them gain greater wisdom and enlightenment. And this is exactly the exciting process in which your unborn baby is involved right now!

I believe that French author, archeologist, and Jesuit priest Pierre Teilhard (1881–1955) was referring to the process of reincarnation when he was quoted as saying, "We are not human beings having a spiritual experience; but, rather, spiritual beings having a human experience."

Once a baby arrives on earth, his soul, or spirit, is no longer a beam or ball of light. At birth, he must surrender to being encapsulated inside a physical body that will sustain him throughout his earthly lifetime. While he is on earth, he is a spiritual being having a human experience. And, like in heaven, he can manifest what he most desires by focusing on a goal. But on earth—*unlike* in heaven—a goal can only be turned into a reality by combining intent, action, faith, and a lot of patience!

Earth is a place we visit because it offers us the adversity we need to evolve, so I refer to the earthly plane as the spiritual boot camp of the universe. Prior to each journey to earth, we must create a specific set of goals to accomplish while there. This means that your unborn baby has already established his agenda, or spiritual blueprint. His plans include: conducting a life's work that will make a difference in other people's lives and help the volatile earthly plane become a better place; resolving certain emotional issues that will allow him to become a more enlightened, wise, and mature individual; and fulfilling spiritual contracts, which involves him acting as both teacher and student with individuals—including you, his mother—who are fellow spiritual beings having a human experience.

Do you realize that you—and your unborn baby—have had *thousands* of prior lifetimes on the earthly plane? This means that you and your unborn baby have traveled back and forth from heaven to earth to be with one another on many occasions. Prevailing over the numerous challenges you've faced throughout all of those journeys is how you have developed into the mature, enlightened beings that you are right now.

It's fascinating to note that Henry Ford, (1863–1947), founder of the Ford Motor Company, was quoted as saying, "I am in exact accord with the belief of Thomas Edison that spirit is immortal, that there is a continuing center of character in each personality. For thirty years I have leaned toward the theory of reincarnation. We are here in life for one purpose—to get experience."

Make no mistake: the transition from heaven to earth requires a tremendous amount of strength, courage, faith, and tenacity—in spite of the fact that your baby will find himself in your loving arms once he is born. You and the soul of your unborn baby are a cohesive team.

Sonya's Story

Throughout my entire pregnancy I have felt very close to my little boy, Travis. We named him after my husband's brother, who passed away years before. I often talk to the baby and can sense his love and connection to me. From early on in the pregnancy I could tell that we were going to make a great team, and my anticipation to meet him grew with each passing day.

During my thirty-fourth week I made an appointment with Julie, a Reiki master and medium, to help me become more calm in preparation for labor and delivery. I also wanted to do some energy work with Travis and make sure he was in the right position and doing everything necessary to prepare for his birth. As we proceeded with the Reiki session, my baby came through and told us that he might need glasses after he was born. He wanted to make me aware that I should pay attention to his eyesight. He also told Julie that he had a kink in his neck, which she was able to alleviate through energy work.

Travis proceeded to show us that he was head down and facing my back, which is the desired position for labor and delivery. He was preparing himself for the big day and told us that he felt very connected to me. Julie informed me that Travis understood that he and I would work together as a team during labor and delivery. Travis told me that my labor would go smoothly and that there would be no major complications. He was very peaceful as he shared this information with us. We were told that he would be guided by his Uncle Travis (my husband's brother) and that his uncle would also be guiding him and protecting him—as he would have protected his own child—all through his life.

I know that the baby has done everything he needs to do in preparation for the big day and that I must remain calm, cool, and collected to do my part. I like thinking of the two of us as a strong team, and I know that we will work together to bring him into this world. My due date is only two weeks away, and I already know that he is a wonderful child. I am so anxious and excited to meet him I could burst!

Truly, it is an exciting journey for each of us to return to the earthly plane. While it is true that all of the "fellow travelers" with whom we'll be interacting have come from heaven just like us, some of them may forget, or develop what I refer to as spiritual amnesia, shortly after they arrive on the earthly plane. This means that they may not remember heaven or the dynamics of their spiritual blueprint.

It requires amazing courage and conviction for your unborn child to journey back to the earthly plane. He realizes that when he is born, he will be completely dependent upon others to feed and clothe him, and provide adequate shelter from the elements. In addition, he knows that it will likely be more than two full years before he can verbally communicate his needs to you and his other caretakers. Each child who chooses you as a parent is trusting that you will rise to the occasion to take care of him and provide the greatest opportunities that will allow him to fulfill his chosen destiny—an awesome and spectacular responsibility!

Prior to becoming a professional channel, I was unconvinced about reincarnation. Although I believed that every human being had a soul, I remained skeptical about an afterlife and the soul's capacity to move back and forth between heaven and earth. But as time went on and I slowly embarked on my spiritual path, I began to question things that had never occurred to me before.

For example, I wondered how Shirley Temple could have begun acting, singing, and dancing before the age of three—like a thirty-year-old seasoned performer. I once read that she had firmly established her career as a Hollywood star by the ripe old age of four!

I'm also fascinated by the legend of the great artist Pablo Picasso. When he was a toddler, in his eagerness to draw, his first spoken word was "pencil." My curiosity then led me to think about all of the other little children throughout history who had been recognized for their prodigious talents.

After I became a professional channel, I asked the guardian angels about this puzzling question and they explained that *earthly skills can only be developed while living on the earthly plane.* Therefore, it may be argued that youngsters who exhibit talents and abilities far beyond their years are living proof that they have existed on the earthly plane before—in previous lives.

Perhaps you've had an experience that caused you to wonder where *your* innate gifts, talents, and abilities originated? For instance, have you ever attempted to do something for the very first time and been surprised that it seemed somehow—familiar? And as you performed this activity, you discovered that you were very good at it right away, as if you were simply picking up where you left off sometime before, in spite of the fact that you *knew* you'd never done it before in your current life? Your baby will experience this too. Every child returning to the earthly plane has his own unique, fully established skills and abilities developed in previous lifetimes on earth.

Once your child is born, his innate gifts, talents, and abilities will shine forth and become quite apparent. When this happens, you're likely to shake your head in amazement and ask your partner, "Where did little Billy *learn* how to do that?" Perhaps he learned those skills in a prior life . . . with you!

Your unborn baby's gifts and talents may start to emerge even *before* he's born, and become perceptible to you, family members, friends—and even strangers—who are sensitive to his presence.

Kaia's Story

I recently attended a lecture in Sedona, Arizona, where I was seated next to a woman who was four months pregnant. As she sat next to me, something extraordinary began to happen. The soul of her unborn baby started to communicate with me.

First, I felt waves of unconditional love flooding my body. It was as if the baby suddenly began to share its energy with me. I was filled with an immense sense of love and peace that emanated from the baby's soul. Next, I felt the joy and playfulness of the soul—which felt distinctively masculine—which conveyed how much he cherished me and what a "joy it was to play with me in this manner on the physical plane."

Finally, the soul began to share his healing energy with me. It felt like sonar or radar waves were coursing through my entire body . . . and I had the impression that he was trying to diagnose whether I needed any healing! It was a distinct *knowing*. After the waves of energy stopped, I felt work going on in my body that involved removing blockages and clearing my physical, emotional, and spiritual energy. As if all of this was not powerful enough, I also felt as if I was carrying this amazing being in my own body.

I was blessed by my interaction with this soul, and I marvel at the gifts he will bring to our planet once he arrives back on physical earthly plane.

When your baby is born, he will possess numerous gifts, talents, and abilities that he developed in prior earthly lives. Likewise, he will also carry certain fears and hesitations that reflect challenges or traumas that he experienced in previous earthly lives. I once had a client who was deathly afraid of water and she had no idea why. When I began to channel, her angels provided a clear picture inside my mind's eye about what had occurred. I "saw" that in her last lifetime, she had died a horrible death as a third class passenger on the ill-fated *Titanic*. During our session, while I described at length what had transpired as I witnessed it in my mind's eye, she cried inconsolably. However, once she understood that she wasn't crazy, and that there was a logical reason for her fear, she was able to move forward—with no more fear of the water.

Possessing this awareness will allow you to be more sensitive to the fears or insecurities your child may exhibit—that he carries with him from experiencing past life trauma—and you'll be able to provide the support and encouragement necessary to help him heal that much faster.

Déjà vu is an intriguing element of reincarnation. Have you ever met someone for the very first time who seemed oddly familiar, as though you somehow already knew the individual, and had an existing trust and affection for them? By contrast, have you ever met someone for the first time and immediately formed an unexpected dislike or distrust of that person for no apparent reason? I've discovered that, while on the earthly plane, we are continually exposed to souls we've known before in other lives, and our immediate reaction to them results from the kind of positive or negative experiences we shared in the past.

Another good example of déjà vu is when an individual visits a place they've never been to before, and yet the surroundings seem surprisingly familiar: *I don't know how, but I'm certain that there is a church around the next corner . . . then a row of houses along a narrow street . . . and a field just beyond that! But I've never been here before . . . so how could I know that?*

Were you aware that you sporadically return to "visit" prior lifetimes in your dreams? Can you recall a dream in which you saw yourself in a different time and place? In the dream, you might have been returning to the scene of a trauma, or to reexamine a violent accident or death, or some type of terrible loss. Past-life dreams can also provide a glimpse back into a time in which you experienced a triumph, such as discovering a life's work that you found thrilling, traveling to exotic far-off places, or enjoying the love of a soul mate and children. You were likely dreaming about a prior life in which you really did those things! Your baby is certain to dream about his past lives, too. Some of these dreams will be very positive and inspiring, as he dreams about exhilarating accomplishments achieved in times gone by. However, if he has healing to do from prior earthly lifetimes, he may experience night terrors.

Night Terrors

There is a phenomenon that occurs so routinely with children under the age of six—at night while they sleep, in the form of dreams—that pediatricians and other healthcare providers refer to it as "night terrors." Night terrors cause a child to wake up from a deep sleep very upset, even to the point of screaming and crying, as if traumatized by some unknown emotional trigger. Although I acknowledge that disruptions in sleep patterns can occur because of a physical ailment or as a result of recently experienced trauma, more often, I believe, it relates to visiting a prior lifetime.

In my experience as a channel, when a parent or grandparent has worriedly inquired about the source of their little one's night terrors, the child's angels have explained that the child—in his dreams—was returning to a prior life on the earthly plane in which a great trauma was suffered. By reliving the episode, the emotional healing process can begin. I have discovered that, following these dreams, a child is able to successfully heal and move on with his current life, unencumbered by the emotional baggage or dysfunction that occurred in a prior lifetime.

Several years ago, the following question was submitted to *Ask Kim*, my monthly advice column:

Dear Kim: I have a question about my grandson Dylan. He wakes up in the middle of the night screaming and crying. My daughter has gotten very little sleep since he was born, and that was more than three years ago. He will only go back to sleep if he is in a recliner in the living room. Is there anything scaring him? To me, he is too old to be waking up and carrying on like this.

Dear Sherry: Dylan's angels tell me that he has been experiencing something commonly referred to as "night terrors." These are past-life dreams that are very clear and vivid; they take him back to prior lifetimes in which he was traumatized or frightened. Your grandson is dreaming about being part of an army in eastern Europe in the Middle Ages. His angels explain that he was a teenage soldier who was captured and then horribly tortured and mutilated. His captor was a man called Vlad the Impaler. Vlad did not come by that nickname because he liked to make shish kebabs on the backyard grill. Look Vlad up online, and you'll see what I mean. It's no wonder that Dylan screams . . . these are not happy little strolls down memory lane that he's taking. His soul is returning to the Middle Ages over and over again, to help him heal from those experiences.

Almost all children have "night terror" dreams, and they sometimes continue for years. My own night terrors, inspired by past-life traumas in Germany's Bergen-Belsen concentration camp, continued until I was about twelve. The important thing to remember is that what Dylan "sees" in his dreams is very real to him—because it actually *did* happen. He needs your support, understanding, and lots of cuddles after such a nightmare.

Sleeping in the recliner makes him feel safer, so why not allow him to do so? It's certainly not ideal, but he needs to feel as safe and secure as possible. Dylan will outgrow the screaming next year—but not the dreams. Plus, he is old enough now to remember how you are responding to his fear and anxiety; so try to react with more tenderness, kindness, and love.

Not all children will experience night terrors. However, if your child has emotional healing to conduct from past-life challenges, he will very likely launch into his healing work very quickly after he first arrives on the earthly plane. That's why small children are predisposed to dream about traumas experienced in past lifetimes. Night terrors happen involuntarily, and usually they are sporadic; the child is not choosing to be naughty, nor does the child enjoy the experience any more than you enjoy your own nightmares. Following one of these dreams, your child will feel very frightened and alone; he will reach out to you for comfort and reassurance.

Possessing this awareness will allow you to be patient and sympathetic should your own child have these common, but sometimes frightening, opportunities to heal. Allow me to suggest that although these dreams are upsetting and disruptive, they are not something to try to avoid. The dreams are your child's soul's way of helping him address and resolve old issues that could potentially cause him difficulties later in his life. The sooner they are resolved, the better!

On April 15, 2004, ABC News *Primetime Live* profiled a true story about a little boy who had past-life memories that were surfacing in his sleep. This is an excerpt of the broadcast:

"Six decades ago, a twenty-one-year-old Navy fighter pilot on a mission over the Pacific was shot down by Japanese artillery. His name might have been forgotten, were it not for six-year-old James Leininger. Quite a few people, including those who knew the fighter pilot, think James is the pilot, reincarnated.

"James's parents, Andrea and Bruce, a highly educated couple, say they are 'probably the people least likely to have a scenario like this pop up in their lives.' But over time, they have become convinced their little son has had a former life. From an early age,

James would play with nothing but planes, his parents say. But when he was two, they said that the planes their son loved began to give him regular nightmares."

"I'd wake him up and he'd be screaming," Andrea told *Primetime Live* co-anchor Chris Cuomo. She said when she asked her son what he was dreaming about, he would say, "Airplane crash on fire, little man can't get out." Andrea says that her mom was the first to suggest James was remembering a past life. Then James's violent nightmares got worse, occurring three or four times a week. Andrea's mother suggested she look into the work of counselor and therapist Carol Bowman, who believes that the dead sometimes can be reborn.

With guidance from Bowman, they began to encourage James to share his memories, and immediately, Andrea says, the nightmares started to become less frequent. James was also becoming more articulate about his apparent past, she said. Bowman said James was at the age when former lives are most easily recalled. "They haven't had the cultural conditioning, the layering over the experience in this life so the memories can percolate up more easily," she said.

Over time, James's parents say he revealed extraordinary details about the life of a former fighter pilot—mostly at bedtime, when he was drowsy. They say James told them his plane had been hit by the Japanese and crashed. Andrea says James told his father he flew a Corsair, and then told her, "They used to get flat tires all the time." Andrea says that James also told his father the name of the boat he took off from, *Natoma,* and the name of someone he flew with, Jack Larson.

After some research, Bruce discovered that *Natoma* and Jack Larson were real. The *Natoma Bay* was a small aircraft carrier in the Pacific. And Larson is living in Arkansas. Bruce became obsessed, searching the Internet, combing through military records, and interviewing men who served aboard the *Natoma Bay*. He said that James told him he had been shot down at Iwo Jima. James had also begun signing his crayon drawings "James 3." Bruce soon learned that the only pilot from the squadron killed at Iwo Jima was James M. Huston Jr. Bruce says James also told him his plane had sustained a direct hit on the engine.

Ralph Clarbour, a rear gunner on a U.S. airplane that flew off the *Natoma Bay*, says his plane was right next to one flown by James M. Huston Jr. during a raid near Iwo Jima on March 3, 1945. Clarbour said he saw Huston's plane struck by anti-aircraft fire. "I would say he was hit head on, right in the middle of the engine," he said. Bruce says he now believes his son had a past life in which he was James M. Huston Jr. "He came back because he wasn't finished with something."

And yet another fascinating detail of the story is that the soul of James M. Huston Jr. once again chose the same name—James—that he had in his last lifetime!

When I was a child, I had horrific nightmares about trains and being locked up. In these dreams, I would find myself hiding under a bed of some kind, and a scary man wearing polished black boots would stride up to where I was concealed. The approach of this man was so terrifying that I would wake up thrashing and crying in my little bed. At the time, in the early 1960s, we lived close to a railroad track. When trains would chug toward our house, I can remember saying to my mother, "All of those poor people!" Puzzled, she would respond, "No, honey, those are freight trains. There are no people on them." But nothing she could say dissuaded me from my knowing that all of those cars held people who were being carried to their doom.

As the dreams continued, they expanded to allow me a complete picture of what had occurred in my past life. I was an eight-year-old Jewish girl living in a small village in France with my mother and father. My beloved father, a member of the French resistance, was often absent. I knew that my mother didn't love me and that I was a burden to her. When the Nazis stormed into our small village, my mother was certain that our home would be searched because of my father's involvement in the Resistance. She told me to open the door when the German soldiers came because she would be hiding upstairs in our attic. Under no circumstances was I to disclose that she was there, or I would be in big trouble! A short time later there was a thunderous knock at the door and shouting in a language I didn't understand. Shaking with fear, I opened the door and the soldiers pushed past me. They ransacked our home while I stood hovering by the front door. A soldier grabbed me by the arm and forced me outside and into the back of a truck with some other families from our village. I was the only child who was alone. The women were crying and holding their children, the men looked fearful and resigned. The truck took us to the train station and we were herded into railroad cars. No one knew where we were headed. The train pulled out of the station and we were locked inside with no food or water. It took days to reach our destination. Children cried with hunger and thirst, while their mothers sang lullabies in a futile attempt to comfort them. Several old people died as they lay on the bottom of the boxcar. The train finally came to a stop and the wide doors were yanked open. We jumped onto the platform and only then did we realize where we had been taken. It was the Bergen-Belsen concentration camp. I died of typhus three months later, hiding under a cot in the medical infirmary where they were conducting medical experiments on children.

As the dreams expanded and I could "see" what I had endured, so many of my fears suddenly made sense. No wonder trains scared me! No wonder I kept seeing those shiny black boots! No wonder I was so afraid of being locked up! No wonder I was hiding! I shared these dreams with my mom; and although she was a devout Catholic at the time, she was very sympathetic about my metaphysical experiences. When I was in elementary school I can remember trudging downstairs some mornings in an exhausted stupor and she would hug me and ask "More Nazi dreams?" It was reassuring to be able to discuss them with her.

The dreams continued until I had finished my healing. Why would I have planned such a terrible experience in that prior life? Because I needed to grow and evolve. In that lifetime, my father taught me about how it felt to be really loved; my mother taught me how it felt to be unwanted, abandoned, and betrayed; and the Nazi's allowed me to experience how it felt to have my security shattered by being forcibly taken from my home, persecuted, abused, starved, and to exist consumed with the fear that I was likely to be murdered or die from an illness at any given moment. My soul had planned wisely. One earthly experience had helped me learn about many issues that might otherwise have taken numerous incarnations. That tragic lifetime instilled in me a profound appreciation of independence and empowerment. The devastating sequence of events with my past-life mother has provided me the courage and strength—in this lifetime—to remove myself from relationships in which I am not valued. The Nazis taught me about sympathy, compassion, and the dire consequences of promoting a judgmental attitude toward others. The Nazis also taught me about appreciating each day as if it were my last. So, experiencing everything I planned in that past life has dramatically helped me evolve and expand to become a more enlightened human being. While the intensity of the experience helped me process and resolve a great many serious, complicated issues all in one incarnation, the other side of the equation was that I was left with a significant amount of healing to do in the next incarnation . . . *this* one! So I chose a mother who would help me by supporting all of the overwhelming healing that I had to conduct from the past, just as your child has chosen *you* to help him or her!

A Doctor's Proof of Reincarnation

Yet another convincing argument for reincarnation is the well-documented hypnotherapy sessions conducted by respected healthcare providers, such as renowned psychotherapist and bestselling author Dr. Brian Weiss, chairman emeritus of psychiatry at the Mount Sinai Medical Center in Miami. Dr. Weiss was shocked when one of his patients—while undergoing hypnosis—began recalling past-life traumas that seemed to hold the key to her nightmares and anxiety attacks. By using past-life therapy, he was able to cure her.

Possessing insight into where you've been and what you've done in past lives helps to explain who you really are *now*, and what you're capable of achieving in this lifetime. Plus, if you choose to experience this special type of hypnosis before or after your children are born, you may have the marvelous, insightful opportunity of revisiting another time and place from the past in which you are able to clearly "see" an interaction between you and your unborn babies!

If you're curious about your spiritual past, or your baby's, consider age-regression hypnotherapy. Check with your local Better Business Bureau, ask someone you trust for a referral, or consider scheduling an appointment with a hypnotherapist who has written a book about it that you've enjoyed.

I believe that by exploring the process of reincarnation, you can more fully foster your child's unique destiny. Whether you are a biological or adoptive parent, you are choosing to be a special conduit through which a new life will be born and nurtured. Your child is arriving to make the earthly plane a better place to live—for his family, friends, and community. Perhaps at some time in his extraordinary life, he will even create positive changes and shifts in the world at large. By believing in your child's talents, abilities, and enlightenment, and through cultivating his positive sense of self and what he can contribute, *you* are acting in the capacity of a guardian angel on the earthly plane. Those of us who are parents are privileged to bear this responsibility.

YOUR CHILD'S DESTINY

I am frequently asked if a child's destiny on the earthly plane is a series of foregone conclusions that are preordained, and therefore not subject to change; or if there is an opportunity for an individual to exercise free will in his decision making. Think of your child's destiny, and your own, as a series of elaborate plans— like a blueprint—that you created while still in heaven and is a kind of spiritual to-do list that you plan to achieve while on earth.

Every individual has his own extensive blueprint that is unique and different from anyone else's. Once you are born, your foundation is laid. Then it is up to you to begin the building process as you make all of the various decisions you face on a daily basis. The universe remains neutral in regard to how and when you build; that is completely up to you. But keep in mind that as you go about the building process, little by little, you're creating your quality of life. You, yourself, created the quality of life you have right now.

Although your baby has a specific destiny that he planned while he was still in heaven, once he returns to the earthly plane, he will have the free will to decide if, how, when, and where he is going to achieve it as he grows up. His guardian angels will assist him, armed with a full understanding of his destiny and all of its different dynamics. In addition, his soul contains a memory bank consisting of everything he has ever done or said in each of his past earthly lives, as well as the blueprint of what he plans to accomplish in this lifetime. This memory bank holds information about his gifts, talents, and abilities—this is the foundation from which he chose his life's work for this lifetime. No one would ever choose a life's work that they were ultimately not capable of achieving. Therefore, you and your unborn baby have chosen your purpose on earth based upon the talents, interests, passions, and skills you developed in prior earthly lives.

Besides being a sophisticated computer, the soul acts as a compass throughout our lives on the earthly plane, providing guidance and direction as each of us searches for the right spiritual path. The soul conveys this insightful information to us through our emotional feelings, rather than logical thought processes.

Speaking of feelings, I've learned—from the information I've received from guardian angels—that true happiness is indeed possible on the earthly plane, and it is achievable by accomplishing three tasks. These tasks, I believe, are the keys to creating remarkably positive changes in your life, as well as allowing you to become a fabulous spiritual mentor for your child.

FIRST TASK: Developing an awareness of your life's work, the issues you need to resolve, and the specifics about your spiritual contracts with others.

Remembering who you are and what you have journeyed to earth to do can create a huge shift in your ability to set appropriate goals and have a sense of meaningful direction. Consider how much easier, simpler, and emotionally rich your life could become if you knew all about your gifts, talents, and abilities—and had a full understanding of what your life's work entailed. You'd be brimming with purpose, initiative, and excitement, which would ultimately lead to a wonderful sense of achievement once you accomplished the various dynamics of your spiritual blueprint.

"How strange is the lot of us mortals!" Albert Einstein, (1879–1955) winner of the Nobel Prize for Physics, once commented. "Each of us is here for a brief sojourn; for what purpose he knows not, though he senses it." Einstein also believed, "If you want to live a happy life, tie it to a goal, not to people or things."

Throughout our entire earthly sojourn, we often struggle to lift the veil of spiritual amnesia that prevents us from building the happiest quality of life possible and contributing as much as we're capable of to our fellow man. As a channel, I've had the privilege of guiding people—through messages from their angels, unborn babies, and departed loved ones—to "remember" exactly what they've come to earth to do and the necessary steps they must take to create true, lasting happiness.

In this regard, I've learned that to develop spiritual awareness, an individual can allow daily life to slowly run its course, and in the process, learn about who she is little by little; or, an individual can simply ask her angels or unborn baby about her destiny, and they can fill her in much faster! In Chapter Five, you'll find my simple step-by-step technique that can allow you, with just a little practice, to tangibly communicate with your unborn baby, guardian angels, and departed family members, if you so desire. When you communicate with them, you can ask about your life's work and other facets of your destiny, which they are sure to know and will be eager to share. The more you develop your self-awareness, the more spiritually enlightened you will become. A channeling session that I conducted recently for a client named Pamela is a good example of how you can build a better quality of life through developing greater self-awareness:

> Kim: I see you're pregnant! Congratulations! What would you like to ask your angels or unborn baby?
>
> Pamela: I want to ask about my career and what I'm going to do professionally after the baby comes. I *hate* the thought of going back to the office after Julia is born . . . but my husband and I need the extra income.
>
> Kim: Your angels tell me that you are *not* in your life's work right now.
>
> Pamela: What does "life's work" mean?
>
> Kim: Life's work refers to the kind of occupation that would make your heart and soul sing, and allow you to make a difference in other peoples' lives.
>
> Pamela: What I'm doing now at the office makes my heart and soul *ache*.
>
> Kim: Your angels tell me that you'd like working from home.
>
> Pamela: I've always wanted to do that—I just haven't been able to figure out how! Maybe I should start a small bookkeeping business?

Kim: Isn't that exactly the kind of work that you're trying to move away from?

Pamela: But that's all I know how to do.

Kim: That's all you now *believe* you know how to do.

Pamela: Huh?

Kim: Your life's work involves being creative, rather than toiling over all of the bookkeeping and accounting details that you currently handle on a daily basis. Have you ever thought of writing?

Pamela: No—I *hate* writing. If you are really speaking with my daughter and angels, wouldn't they already know that?

Kim: Your baby, Julia, says that you hate writing *letters* and *reports*.

Pamela: That's all I do every day—and I'm sick of it!

Kim: Your life's work involves a completely different kind of writing. Julia says that you're supposed to be writing children's books.

Pamela: Children's books? I wouldn't have the faintest clue how to go about that!

Kim: You can't be confident about something you haven't done yet.

Pamela: Well . . . that's true.

Kim: Julia's birth will be the catalyst for the books. You're going to name one of the characters after your daughter.

Pamela: Writing books sounds crazy to me.

Kim: Your books will make a big difference in the lives of children around the world. When you're recovering from Julia's birth, your angels want you to sit at the computer and begin the first book. Your destiny is to write a series of stories based upon characters that include a big group of farm animals with distinct personalities. In the first book, they're going to help heal an injured baby moose.

Pamela: Oh my gosh! I can't believe it! That's the story that keeps running through my head—like a song that won't stop playing! I've been wondering where it was coming from.

Kim: Julia and your angels have been sharing it in order to help you get into your life's work.

Pamela: It's really a cute story! I have recurring dreams about it. Last weekend, I almost sat down in front of my computer to write it all down . . . but then I thought that was a crazy idea.

Kim: Then you already *know* what to do.

Pamela: I do?

Kim: Do you believe in reincarnation?

Pamela: I think so.

Kim: You've been an author in a number of your past lives—so there is no way that you cannot do this! Consider your past-life experience as the foundation from which you will work in this lifetime. You'd *love* writing these whimsical stories! And as an author, you'd have lots of wiggle room with your daily schedule to accommodate Julia's needs, plus you'll earn a lot more money than you do at your current job. You won't have to kiss anyone's posterior to get time off, and you'll be making a difference in the lives of the children who read your books! How wonderful is *that?*

Pamela: So channeling is this simple? It's like reorganizing—

or reframing—a lot of what I already *know*? Like the moose story that keeps running through my head? So you're telling me that those dreams have actually happened for a reason?

Kim: Yes! And as you practice your own channeling, the information will flow faster from your unborn baby and your angels and seem more tangible. You'll have more intuitive dreams, too.

Pamela: This explains so much. I'd love to work from home! And perhaps the books might help children develop faith in themselves as they learn from the animal characters that I keep seeing in my dreams? I just have to stop being so negative and afraid when I think about money or doing something new.

Kim: Now you're getting the picture. You have a very important purpose on the earthly plane.

Pamela: I just have to muster the faith that I can actually do this. The thought of it—*all* of it—makes me very happy and peaceful inside.

Kim: Keep in mind that you would never have chosen a destiny that was too hard for you to accomplish.

Pamela: My baby is suddenly kicking like crazy!

Kim: I am hearing her say, "I'm proud of you, Mommy! Let's go have lunch!"

Pamela: (laughter) Now I have something concrete to work toward—like a mission. I've never felt a real sense of purpose before. Just knowing that I won't have to stay in an office job forever makes my heart and soul sing!

SECOND TASK: The second task includes accomplishing your agenda by mustering the faith and conviction to be who you are and to take a stand on behalf of your convictions.

Winston Churchill is a wonderful example of someone who had the courage to withstand a blistering torrent of negativity and remain steadfast in his convictions. During the mid-1930s, he became increasingly troubled over the fact that Germany was manufacturing arms at a staggering rate and was rapidly fortifying its military. When he shared his concern with Parliament, he was shouted down as an alarmist and was told, in essence, to keep his paranoid ramblings to himself. But he mustered the courage to remain steadfast in his position, amidst a furor of public criticism. A few years later, when his concerns became a reality, his peers offered him the post of prime minister. By that time, it was already almost too late, as Germany had begun plans to swallow Europe and was headed for war with Britain. However, Churchill prevailed and triumphed because of the strength of his resolute determination and his refusal to give up.

Few of us will be called upon to save our country as he was; but each one of us has chosen a destiny to make some kind of difference in the world. Are you making yours? Or are you allowing others to force you in a direction that does not make your heart and soul sing? Perhaps you dream about a certain career, but your family wouldn't approve? Perhaps you have come to embrace a new spiritual philosophy that wouldn't be popular with friends or family? Perhaps you understand that if you set boundaries and stand up for yourself, certain people will become angry or hurt, and shut you out? Then so be it! You have no control over the decisions other people make—but you do have control over your own choices.

Be a parent who leads by example. This is a perfect time to release the need or desire to have other people's endorsement or approval of what you want to do. You might be surprised to learn that the majority of people fail to create a life that makes their heart and soul sing because they lack the approval or support of others. Muster the courage to make the choices that most appeal to you. Declare yourself—regardless of what others think or how they'll react—and you'll be on your way to true happiness, and watch your child grow up to be an individual who does the same.

THIRD TASK: Learning to bloom where you are presently planted, and valuing every moment of your life.

This means that no matter *what* is going on in your life, you can maintain a joyful existence simply by making that *choice*. In other words, when something occurs that is upsetting, hurtful, angering, depressing, frightening, or stressful, you can choose not to allow the situation to disrupt your emotional equilibrium. "Blooming" where you are—no matter *what* is going on around you—is, admittedly, far easier in theory than in practice. Think of a little clock sitting on a bedside table. A storm could be raging outside, but inside, the clock on the nightstand continues its tick . . . tick . . . tick, completely unaffected. Children are wonderful bloomers. French author Jean de La Bruyère (1645–1696) once said: "Children have neither past nor future; they enjoy the present, which very few of us do."

Since their births, my son and daughter have always taught me through their example very valuable lessons about blooming. However, it took a natural disaster for me to finally understand what it meant.

We live in Texas, eighty miles from Galveston, which is located on the Gulf of Mexico. The Gulf Coast is vulnerable to hurricanes every year from May through November. In September 2008, Hurricane Ike hit the coast, causing so much damage that Texas Governor Rick Perry's office was quoted as saying, "Hurricane Ike will likely go down in history as the most costly and destructive storm ever to hit Texas."

As Hurricane Ike approached landfall, I was worrying about protecting my children. I asked my angels about what we could expect, and they assured me that no one in the family would be hurt. They went on to say that we would sustain heavy rains and strong winds, but there would be no flooding in our area. In preparation, while my husband hurriedly nailed plywood over all of the windows to protect them from flying debris, I assembled candles, flashlights, nonperishable foods, and filled bathtubs and buckets full of water to use after the storm so we could bathe and flush toilets.

The night of the storm, I hunkered down in the den with my husband and two children in our sleeping bags. Anticipating that the situation might get a little scary, I tried to make a game out of it by suggesting to my seven- and eight-year-old that we were camping and experiencing an adventure like the Swiss Family Robinson. I was determined to remain positive and unafraid in order to help my children cope with whatever was going to come.

It wasn't long before the winds picked up and heavy rain began to fall. We heard the mechanical groan of the neighborhood transformer shutting down, and we lost power. We huddled together in the darkness as the rains increased and the winds became alarming.

With each mighty gust of wind, I began to hear something outside over the terrific roar of the storm that I couldn't identity, and it was extremely unnerving. I can only describe it as a very loud creaking door. With the next gust of wind, I heard the noise again, and then a CRACK! was followed by a BOOM! The towering, majestic pine trees that surrounded our home were being ripped apart by the ferocious winds, creating the creaking-door sound. Huge tree tops and massive limbs began to fall outside all around us, so heavy they shook the ground when they landed.

At the height of the storm, the torrential rain was so explosive that I was certain our house was going to flood. I heard another loud, alarming creaky-door sound, and then CRACK! BOOM! A huge pine tree had fallen into the second floor of our house! My husband and I scrambled to the second floor and then up inside the attic, where, pelted by the driving rains, I assisted while he created funnels from plastic lawn bags, and nailed them over the gaping holes in the roof to guide the heavy rainwater into pots, pans, and other containers that we could quickly grab.

After that was done, I ran back downstairs to my children. My mind was racing! Despite what my angels had told me earlier about our safety, and my determination to remain positive and unafraid, I had become crazy with fear. The reality of our situation was that although the house could provide shelter from the rain, it was no match for one of the pine trees. If a big enough tree fell upon the roof directly above us, it could easily slam through to the second floor—and then through the first floor ceiling—and kill us! We didn't have a basement or any inner rooms, except for the tiny pantry. There was nowhere to take the children that offered significant protection from the trees, and it was a terrible, helpless feeling.

Inexplicably, my seven-year-old daughter Megan had fallen fast asleep in spite of the storm. But my son Flynn was terrified. He asked what would happen if a tree fell into the part of the house where we sat cowering, which was quickly becoming a realistic possibility. I guessed that he was sensing my feelings, which he often does. I looked into his big brown eyes and knew what I had to do. I had to lie. Holding him close, I promised that I would never allow anything to hurt him or Megan. I felt horribly guilty making that promise, knowing that I had absolutely no control over what would happen next! With each powerful gust of wind, the trees creaked, snapped, and fell. I held Flynn in my arms as the storm continued to rage all night long.

Although we sustained more damage from limbs and tree tops falling onto the roof, we remained safe and uninjured; and thankfully, no rising water had come into the house. The heavy winds finally died down, and all that was left of Ike was a penetrating rain that fell throughout the following day.

The next morning, as soon as there was enough light, we opened the back door to peer outside and assess the damage. The yard looked like a war zone. Downed trees and limbs were everywhere. The kids began to cry when they saw their sturdy wooden swing set and play house laying in pieces amid all of the other debris. Our home had withstood the storm, but we had no electricity or water, and temperatures that day were expected to climb into the nineties—with equal levels of humidity.

We drank bottled water and flushed toilets with the buckets of water that I had collected before the storm. My husband, a true hurricane veteran from his years in Louisiana, was stoic, optimistic, and seemingly unfazed. I, however, had been utterly traumatized by the experience. My babies could have been killed!

Although we had intermittent cell phone power, there was no landline telephone service. We were almost completely cut off from the outside world. Needing a brief respite from the depressing situation at home, we decided to carefully explore the area. In our minivan we inched our way around downed trees; dangling power lines; roofing, fence, and signage debris; and the toppled telephone poles that littered the streets. Other homes had sustained damage far worse than ours. In the aftermath of the storm, gas stations, convenience stores, banks, grocery stores, restaurants, and schools were closed, and eerily dark and empty. Many of them had also sustained significant damage. It was a very sobering sight.

Back home, we discovered that a bad smell was already coming from inside the refrigerator. Unfortunately, we did not own a generator, so we had to throw away all of our perishable food. The heat inside the house became so oppressive that we couldn't sleep. We ate crackers, apples, and peanut butter at every meal, happy to have them. By candlelight, we took sponge baths in the bathtub with cold buckets of water. Because rainwater had accumulated in different spots in the attic before we could nail the plastic sheeting, we had seepage through the ceilings of the upstairs bath, as well as the living and dining rooms on the first floor. Drywall fell to the floor in wet pieces, soaking the wall-to-wall carpet. The foul odor of mold and mildew began to permeate the house.

Several days after the storm, we still had no power, telephone service, or water. Although it was late at night, Flynn asked if the family could play bingo. We couldn't really sleep because of the heat and humidity, so I reluctantly agreed. Feeling traumatized and very depressed, I wasn't in the mood to play a game. The kids eagerly assembled the lantern and the game pieces on the kitchen table, and the four of us took our seats in the heat and the semidarkness.

"Aaaah, this is the life!" said my son, with a self-satisfied smile.

I just stared back at him, unable to comprehend what he meant. "What do you *mean?*" I asked with astonishment.

"I'm having a great time!" he announced.

"Me too!" said Megan with a grin.

"But . . . *how?*" I asked them. "After the ordeal we've just been through?"

"Mom—that was *days* ago!" replied Megan. "Except for our swing set, we're okay! And we don't have to go to school!"

I stared back at her dumbly.

"Look at all of the family time that we have now!" Flynn pointed out. "Playing bingo by camp light, sleeping on the floor in our sleeping bags, doing man's work cleaning up the yard, cold baths like an army guy, and peanut butter and crackers for breakfast, lunch, and dinner! This is the best time I've ever had!"

"Yeah!" exclaimed Megan. "Mommy . . . you have to turn your brain off! You're being negative! It's an adventure, like the Swiss Family Robinson . . . remember? *We're* having fun! Why aren't *you*?"

I realized that the universe—and my children—were providing just the practice I needed to really learn how to "bloom," regardless of what was going on around me. At that moment, my cell phone rang. My brother, Mike, was calling to tell me that Brennan's Restaurant—a historic Houston landmark where, on numerous occasions, we had celebrated special events—had burned to the ground in the storm. Much worse, a man and his little girl had taken refuge there during the hurricane and had been severely burned. It was not known if they were going to survive their injuries.

What a stunning reality check! As Mike and I said our goodbyes, I gazed at my husband and two children, who were laughing, teasing one another about the game, and obviously enjoying the moment. Suddenly, I understood what "blooming" really meant. Instead of choosing to focus on all of the negative things that had just happened—which I had no power to change—I shifted my focus to all of the things I had to be grateful for.

THREE

DEVELOPING AN AWARENESS OF YOUR BABY'S CHOSEN LIFE'S PATH

Chapter Profile: Are you curious about your baby's destiny? He's already chosen his life's work and the issues that he intends to resolve. This chapter reveals all of the choices he had to make before returning to the earthly plane for his upcoming lifetime—with you!

When a soul in heaven wants to improve itself, how does it go about the transition process? Try to visualize your baby in heaven right now. He yearns to expand his enlightenment and has made the courageous decision to embark on yet another earthly sojourn. From his safe home in heaven, he begins to make a series of exciting, intricate plans that will shape his destiny and form the spiritual blueprint of what he hopes to achieve during his upcoming life with you.

The two biggest decisions a soul has to make involve his life's purpose and the emotional issues he plans to resolve. Those two dynamics comprise the foundation of his spiritual blueprint, but in very different ways. By addressing and resolving certain key issues, he will be benefiting *himself* by developing greater enlightenment, wisdom, and maturity. Through performing a particular life's work, he will have the opportunity to benefit *others* on the earthly plane, as the epicenter of his own positive ripple effect.

Only after he has chosen his life's work and the emotional issues he will attempt to address will all of the other details of his life's path, including gender, name, family of origin, physical appearance, and so on, fall into place.

LIFE'S WORK

If you are currently expecting, your baby has already chosen his life's work. Isn't that *exciting*? In fact, every human being on the earthly plane has planned a specific life's work, including you! But how does one go about making such an important decision?

Souls typically gravitate toward the type of work for which they've had an affinity in prior earthly lifetimes. The life's work we choose is certain to result in spiritual, emotional, and mental fulfillment. Because of this, a soul would never choose a kind of work that he would not be successful in achieving. When I conduct private sessions, clients ask about the nature of their life's work more than any other question. When I reveal specifics about what they are here on the earthly plane to accomplish, often the individual will gasp and respond, "What! Can I *do* that? I'd love to, but I don't know if I'm capable!"

What's more, a soul often continues to choose the same kind of life's purpose again and again; only the *method* by which it conducts the work will shift from lifetime to lifetime.

For example, a soul that enjoys healing may have worked as a doctor in the Middle Ages, healing victims of the plague with flower essences, then returned for another earthly lifetime to work as a doctor in colonial America, healing victims of smallpox with leeches, followed by a lifetime as a surgeon operating on soldiers from the front lines in WWI, and in the present day, works as an orthopedic surgeon in modern-day London, devoting his time to replacing arthritic hips and knees with technologically advanced prosthetic joints.

Souls that gravitate toward the performing and creative arts may have been a poet in the time of Jesus, an actor performing Shakespeare in the Middle Ages, an artist during the Renaissance, then an opera singer in the 1800s, and now an author of children's books.

Other souls may have an affinity for public service. A soul could have chosen to be a diplomat during the reign of Elizabeth I, a sympathetic judge during the Spanish Inquisition, an activist working to free the slaves in antebellum America, an inventor during the Industrial Revolution, and now a member of parliament, fighting for funds to feed the poor.

An intrepid ship's captain who sailed a merchant vessel on uncharted seas to transport silks, spices, and precious stones during the Renaissance may now be a helicopter pilot who ferries donated organs to medical centers for lifesaving transplants.

There are other souls that love to work with the soil as farmers, ranchers, cattlemen, or who own vineyards filled with grapes or olives while they are residing on the earthly plane.

Individuals who enjoy the military often repeat those experiences. General George S. Patton believed that he had past lifetimes on earth as a soldier and spoke openly about it. While he was a young soldier in France during World War I, he wrote to his mother: "I wonder if I could have been here before. As I drive up the Roman road the Theater seems familiar—perhaps I headed a legion up that same white road . . . I passed a chateau in ruins which I possibly helped escalade in the Middle Ages. There is no proof nor yet any denial. We were, we are, and we will be." Perhaps that was why he so fearlessly prevailed during World War II—since developing combat strategies was so familiar to him?

Athletic ability is also echoed from life to life. An individual who participated in the early Olympic games could have been reborn as an Olympian in other incarnations. Perhaps some of the professional athletes today have followed these patterns in past earthly sojourns? Typically, a soul will choose a kind of life's purpose that will allow it to carry on from where it left off in a prior life, seeking to make a mark on the earthly plane and leaving it a better place. Once back on earth, each soul is at the epicenter of its own ripple effect, creating currents of positive shifts that will impact fellow travelers at the level of which it is capable.

In this regard, a soul revisiting earth may choose to raise a family and remain in the same community in which it was born for an entire lifetime, or it could decide to impact the world at large, creating positive change that transcends political philosophies, geographic borders, and religious beliefs . . . like Mother Teresa, Helen Keller, Michelangelo, Thomas Edison, or Clara Barton.

Regardless of the size of the impact it plans to make while on earth, each soul has the same opportunity to develop greater wisdom, maturity, and enlightenment so that its time on earth is wisely invested for itself—and others!

EMOTIONAL ISSUES TO RESOLVE

Once your baby has chosen his *life's purpose* for his upcoming earthly lifetime, which is the special way in which he will contribute to the lives of others, he must then review all of his outstanding *emotional issues* to determine how he is going to build greater wisdom, enlightenment, and maturity to benefit himself— in order to make the earthly journey as successful as possible. For instance, if your baby is planning a life's work in the performing or creative arts, such as painting, acting, singing, dancing, composing, or writing, the issues he may need to resolve could include:

Risk-taking: because these professions are not typically considered secure

Following the dictates of his heart and soul: choosing a particular profession even if he does not receive the endorsement or approval from family or friends who might consider his choice frivolous

Patience and perseverance: because it may take many years for him to become a success

Learning to bloom where he is currently planted: mustering the courage and resolute determination to stay his course and refuse to give up in the face of financial difficulties and self-doubt in the years that unfold before he becomes a success

Faith in his ability: refusing to give up even when others criticize or don't understand his talent

While still in heaven, most souls are extremely optimistic about what they believe is possible for them to address once they are back on earth, so they set a rigorous emotional agenda that usually commences at birth, or in very early childhood, to allow the soul to best utilize all of its precious time on earth. Since the entire purpose of returning to earth is to evolve and help other fellow travelers do the same, every period in the upcoming earthly journey is jam-packed with emotional work. So when you wonder why you've been bombarded by one challenge right after another, now you know that you actually planned it that way!

There is no better time to address your own issues than when you are expecting. In doing so, you will be able to immediately improve your quality of life and teach your child how to do the same as you lead by example. Keep in mind that some issues can be worked through very quickly. Your work will truly be the gift that keeps on giving because you'll have created a much better existence. In addition, when your child faces his own issues, you can apply this newfound awareness to assist him with his work!

GENDER

After your baby has chosen his life's work and the issues he plans to address, he will decide whether he is going to be male or female. This choice will be determined by your baby's assessment of which gender would allow him the greatest opportunities to achieve his life's work and resolve his chosen issues. For that reason, a soul will frequently shift genders from lifetime to lifetime on the earthly plane, allowing it to develop a *balance* between the male and female energies.

For instance, in the metaphysical community, it is believed that each gender has numerous telltale traits. Male energy is considered to be courageous, decisive, physically strong, curious, independent, empowered, analytical, practical, and risk-taking. Female energy is thought of as sensitive, creative, intuitive, patient, understanding, emotionally strong, whimsical, persevering, gentle, and nurturing.

You might be thinking that you have qualities of both genders. That is correct! Because you have lived lifetimes as both a male and a female, you have retained many of these characteristics—even as you choose a specific gender with every lifetime you live.

As a result of returning numerous times to the earthly plane, each soul has the wonderful opportunity to experience life from both the male and female perspective, and it develops the vital balance that depicts true enlightenment. So, if your baby is a boy, you will have the opportunity—as his mother, a woman—to learn even more about male energy beyond what you've already experienced in your previous male lifetimes.

Becky's Story

I had a *knowing*, while I was pregnant, about the fact that I was going to have a boy. So I wrote my unborn son a letter to tell him about all of the things I hoped and wished for him when he arrived.

What amazed me was that when I was a little girl, I had been an only child who had always played with other girls. I had never been exposed to boy "stuff" like sports, playing with trucks, or climbing trees. I didn't have the faintest idea how to play with a little boy. I guess I had lost sight—or spiritually forgotten—all of the male lifetimes I had before!

I actually fretted over whether I was really the best mom for this child. One day during the pregnancy I came to the realization that my life was going to change completely anyway . . . so I chose not to worry anymore! My son is my only child, and one quality that I have learned from him is an appreciation of what it is to be a boy and a man, as well as some of the emotions and experiences of males that I would not have known had he not chosen me as his mother. It is one thing to be a man's wife; however, watching my darling son Aaron grow up provided me with a completely different perspective of the male experience.

While you might have a particular gender preference, your unborn baby chooses his own gender. What's interesting is that you may be sensing the gender of your child through the bonding that is taking place while the baby is still in utero. If your baby is planning on being a girl, you might start longing for all things frilly and pink. If your child is going to be a boy, you might find yourself instinctively shopping for trucks and building blocks—even before you start "showing" in your first trimester.

Whether she is a biological or adoptive mother, a woman often starts to visualize her baby as a certain gender because that is what the baby is communicating to her. Mothers often start nesting and fantasizing about feeding their newborn, what songs they'll sing to the baby, what books they'll share, and other intimate bonding activities that will be enjoyed once the child arrives. When the little one is finally born and the doctor shouts, "It's a girl!" or "It's a boy!" the mother's reaction is often, *I knew it! I felt it! Just what I wanted!*

However, there *can* be surprises in regard to gender—even for the most intuitive women! First, let's say that your baby does not tell you what his or her gender is going to be, but you know that you're sensing either distinctly male or female energy from the baby. Remember that in this day and time, many souls are a combination of both male and female energies because of the many trips they've previously made to the earthly plane—as both genders. Perhaps in past lives, the child coming to you now has come to you before, and always as a girl. So it is likely that her energy would feel female to you, in spite of the fact that "she" had chosen to be a boy this time around.

Let me give you another example: although I'm a girly-girl, I also have lots of great male energy. I can't pick up the front end of a car, but there are few things that I have to ask my husband or brother to help me with. Plus, I adore doing male-oriented things with my son, like our annual mother-son outing to the Wings Over Houston Air Show. Consequently, it is possible that if I were now living in heaven—as a spirit—and a woman became pregnant with me, my energy might feel masculine to her.

I've also learned in my channeling sessions that there could be a shift in gender because there was a sudden change in birth order. For example, unborn babies commonly do what I refer to as "jockeying for position." This means that as children hover around their chosen birth mother, they decide who goes first, second, and so on. The souls determine their birth order. Certain personalities want to come first, like my son Flynn. Other souls prefer being a middle child, or the baby, like my daughter, Megan.

There are instances in which a particular child makes all of his plans in regard to returning to the earthly plane, and then decides—right before the conception—to change the order of his birth. This happens frequently. And you, very likely, will continue to interact with this unborn child, who is still planning on coming to you . . . simply at a different time than when he had originally shared with you in dreams, intuitive feelings, or through messages conveyed in tangible conversations. Therefore, as you communicate with your unborn baby, consider asking about whether he or she has had a change of plans in regard to order of birth.

Spiritual Contracts

Once we decide upon our life's work, issues, and gender, we connect with other souls planning to return to the earthly plane who could help us with our spiritual agenda. A spiritual contract is a promise or commitment that we make with other souls who we plan to interact with sometime during our upcoming earthly life. The interaction might last a lifetime, or just a few minutes. The connection will last long enough for the promise to be fulfilled.

You have a very significant spiritual contract with your unborn baby. He has specifically chosen you to be a vitally important teacher and mentor. Through your efforts, he can evolve into his full potential and contribute what he is capable of on the earthly plane. Imagine your unborn baby at the epicenter of his own ripple effect. In his upcoming lifetime with you, he will contribute to the lives of others and leave the earthly plane a better place than how he found it. Remember that he has chosen you as a mother because he trusts that you will nurture his self-worth, sense of awareness, and confidence . . . which are the key components that will allow him to achieve his special spiritual blueprint.

Furthermore, the spiritual contract between you and your child works both ways. Your unborn baby is coming into your life not only as a student, but as a teacher for you. Through parenting this extraordinary little being, you're going to discover so much more about who you are, what you're capable of, and even how your priorities will dramatically shift and change. For instance, when I'm worried or concerned about being able to accomplish a new challenge, I just remember that I birthed a nine-pound, four-ounce baby, and suddenly I'm Super Woman! I tell myself that I can do anything!

In addition, you'll discover that some of the things that currently frustrate you, or that you find stressful, won't have anywhere near the same impact—because you have the privilege of loving and nurturing the precious little being who depends on you for his very life. Once you've had your baby, nearly everything else takes a back seat, and you'll find yourself not sweating the small stuff connected with work, money, friends, or family members.

With the help of this book, you can ask your unborn baby about all of the marvelous lessons you are meant to help him with so that you are fully prepared before he arrives. Plus, you can ask him about the lessons he is going to teach you.

For example, one of the reasons I chose my mother is that I knew she would help me with three of my most challenging issues: independence, empowerment, and self-esteem. And by golly, she did! Throughout my childhood I saw her choosing to remain in an abusive marriage—always fraught with terrible money problems—because she was too frightened to go off on her own as a single parent with three children. I learned by watching her. Little by little, I became self-reliant and assertive so I would never feel emotionally trapped by financial neediness or fear like she was. Ironically, she constantly told *me*, "There's nothing you can't achieve!" and I took that to heart. To this day, when someone tells me that something can't be done, or that I don't have the ability to accomplish a certain goal, I remember her faith in me and it always bolsters my confidence.

In Thomas Edison's early life, a teacher contacted his mother to pick him up from school and try to educate him at home because, in his opinion, young Thomas wasn't bright enough to keep up with the other kids. Filled with indignation, his mother escorted Thomas out of school and proceeded to teach him at home. Had his mother failed to rise to the occasion for her son, it is possible that his life would have taken a very different course. In fact, he was quoted as saying, "My mother was the making of me. She was so true, so sure of me; and, I felt I had something to live for, someone I must not disappoint."

For a moment, consider all of the people you have met throughout your life. Whether you've been aware of it or not, you've shared prior earthly incarnations with all of them. What's more, you've had predestined spiritual contracts with many of these individuals. In these special relationships, we act as student and teacher for one another.

So how do we form these contracts? While still in heaven, we gravitate toward other souls who have picked issues to resolve that dovetail perfectly with our own. If you are going to work on learning to set boundaries with others, you'll form a contract with someone who is controlling and dictatorial. Sparks will fly throughout the relationship, but you'll both have the opportunity to learn from one another, if you *choose* to do so. Perhaps you have an issue with patience. You'd choose to engage with someone who is a procrastinator. Or maybe you have an issue being able to say "no!" comfortably. Then you'd plan to have an interaction with someone who is selfish and takes advantage of others to provide you with a lot of practice standing up for yourself. In each of these relationships, you have the opportunity to resolve an issue and become a more mature and enlightened individual. Therefore, the faster you work through an issue, the sooner a difficult person moves out of your lives.

Besides spiritual contracts that are destined to have confrontational, hurtful, or annoying consequences, we also plan to interact with others who have promised to be supportive, encouraging, and loving, such as a soul mate relationship. Still others have promised to be facilitators, mentors, or healers for us. We plan to meet each of the individuals with whom we have a spiritual contract in a specific timeframe to allow us the greatest advantage of actually addressing an issue. Consider all of the relationships you've had in the past. What do you think you were destined to learn from them?

Unfortunately, complications arise when an individual fails to honor his spiritual contracts. Imagine that you go on a job interview with someone who has a spiritual contract to be a mentor and facilitator for you. Instead of hiring you for the job, he turns you down, failing to recognize that he was supposed to be of help. Imagine that you go in for a necessary surgery with a physician who has a spiritual contract to help you heal—and because of drinking to excess the night before, he botches the operation. Imagine that you meet someone who is supposed to be a soul mate for you and offer you a lifelong heart, mind, body and soul relationship—but, instead, breaks off the romance. These unfortunate scenarios happen all the time on the earthly plane. Since we have absolutely zero control over other people's choices, it is imperative that we recognize what *our* particular spiritual contracts entail with others and honor those promises—regardless of whether they are reciprocated.

When you meet someone new, remember that you were brought together for an important spiritual reason, and in the exact time frames in which you were both ready to be teacher and student for one another. If there is a spiritual contract, you'll feel a pull toward that individual, or a connection that definitely registers on your intuitive radar screen.

In order to figure out specifics about *why* you were brought together with a certain individual, you can allow the relationship to unfold and learn from the issues that eventually emerge between you; or you could speed up the process by simply asking your guardian angels or unborn baby about why a particular person has come into your life. I provide my simple, step-by-step technique in Chapter Five that can have you channeling proficiently with just a little practice. I encourage you to get into the habit of asking your angels and unborn baby about everyone you meet. This will allow you to better honor all of the contracts that you committed to before you were reborn on the earthly plane.

Take a moment to recall the family that surrounded you when you were a child. Who provided you with the greatest level of adversity? Those individuals were some of your best teachers. What did you learn from them? Who supported and encouraged you? What did you learn from them? Some people with whom we interact have the spiritual responsibility to teach us what *to do*, while others have the spiritual responsibility to teach us what *not to do*.

Planning the relationships that we expect to impact us throughout the course of our lifetimes on earth is incredibly labor-intensive and time-consuming; you went to a lot of trouble to plan these interactions—just like your unborn baby is doing now! If you remember how someone subjected you to hurt, disappointment, anger, abuse, or neglect in your early years, it is very likely that you deliberately chose that individual to jump-start your ability and desire to mature and evolve. In fact, those individuals actually rose to the occasion for you, just as you anticipated!

Each one of our early relationships is vitally important in regard to fine-tuning a stronger sense of self, elevating our self-worth, cultivating a far more resilient level of confidence (especially when we're faced with new challenges), and providing the perfectly calibrated inspiration to achieve the spiritual agenda we've set for ourselves. You would not be the person you are today without the help and guidance of all of the people with whom you interacted in your childhood. And your unborn baby would not be able to reach his full potential without you—and all of his other spiritual teachers.

FAMILY OF ORIGIN

Now a soul is ready to choose his all-important family of origin. This includes birth parents, adoptive parents (if the soul is planning to be raised by someone other than his biological parents), siblings, and members of the extended family such as grandparents, aunts, uncles, cousins, and close family friends.

Lori's Story

My six-year-old, Oliver, was in first grade and each of his classmates had made a turkey art project for Thanksgiving. On each of the turkey's feathers was a note of thanks. He said he was thankful for his mom, dad, sisters, baby brother, etc. At student conference time, Mrs. Wilkstrom, his teacher, congratulated us on our new baby. When I expressed surprise, she showed us the feather on the turkey that read "baby brother." My husband and I looked at each other in confusion and then chuckled in amusement, knowing that Oliver did not have a baby brother, only two younger sisters.

Shortly thereafter, my daughters, three-year-old Saige and five-year-old Epiffany, asked if we could have another baby. At this time, I was fifty pounds overweight and not very enthusiastic about another pregnancy. I believed that our family was complete with three children. Then my husband mentioned that it would be great to have another baby. I still resisted, saying that I needed to lose at least twenty pounds before I could carry another pregnancy; plus, our new home was not finished yet. The whole family kept asking, and I kept resisting and taking my birth control pills. But finally, I agreed to try.

After only three months, our fourth child was conceived. I really think that he chose our family. At the time, I was busy taking care of the three we had, working full time, building a new house, trying to recover from six years of sleep deprivation, and trying to lose the baby weight from the previous three pregnancies! So I believe that the baby's only means of communicating was through his future siblings.

I still find it a miracle that a three- and five-year-old would suggest, "Momma, have another baby . . . we want another baby."

And how would a six-year-old know to be grateful for a baby brother before he was even conceived?

I am so thankful for our fourth child, Liam. He was conceived in complete love and still reflects that in his essence every day. I am blessed for all of my children.

Consider how different your baby's life would have been if, instead of choosing you as a parent in his upcoming earthly lifetime, he had decided to be born inside the caste society of India as an untouchable? Or if he had chosen to be born inside the British royal family as the next in line to the throne? Or into a modest farm family in rural Kansas? Or into an affluent ranching family in Argentina? Imagine how different his life would have been had he chosen to become the child of a celebrity, president, or prime minister?

It's fascinating to note that being born into extreme wealth or extreme poverty does not always create greater—or lesser—chances of developing enlightenment. We've all heard stories about individuals rising to success regardless of the challenges of their birth or the circumstances of their early lives. In fact, some of the most inspiring stories about people who have achieved a very impressive destiny have begun their lives in very modest financial circumstances, or in families where they were not supported, nurtured, understood, or celebrated for who they were.

NAME

One of the benefits of bonding with your child before birth is to allow you to become familiar with his likes and dislikes—including name preference. If you are pregnant right now, your child is probably already communicating what he would prefer his name to be.

Susan's Story

When I became pregnant with my second child, my husband and I decided that we wanted to be completely surprised by the baby's sex when I gave birth. I had picked out a girl's name, but I was having a tough time trying to pick out a name for a boy. I began to believe that I was going to have another girl for that reason . . . and my whole family thought I was carrying a girl, too.

At about my eighth month, I had a dream that I was driving through a charming old town lined with red brick buildings adorned with hanging flower baskets on the windows. It had a very nostalgic feeling. The town seemed to be empty and I wondered where everyone had gone.

Suddenly, in my rear view mirror, I could see that a boy of about eight had ridden out onto the street a couple of blocks behind me on a Radio Flyer bike. I stopped and he waved at me. As I turned around to drive toward him, he suddenly swiveled, and I knew that he wanted to show me the nameplate under the back of his bicycle seat that read "Eric."

In a playful and mischievous way, he started peddling away from me very quickly, looking over his shoulder and grinning at me, waving for me to keep up. I woke up shortly afterward and told my husband that I was convinced our new child had just introduced himself to us.

When he was born, hearing "It's a boy!" was indescribably thrilling. My son and I were immediately bonded, and I instinctively knew that Eric and I had been together in many lifetimes. We are still very close, and I seem to know what he is thinking before anyone else. Eric is now eight years old and the spitting image of the boy in my dream.

If, on the other hand, a parent forces an *unwanted* name on a baby, sooner or later the child will typically choose to go by an abbreviation, initials, a nickname, or another name altogether.

In 1882, a baby girl was born into a prominent Austin family. She would grow up to be known as the "First Lady of Texas" and become one of the most generous philanthropists of her time. Believe it or not, her parents gave her the unfortunate name of Ima Hogg—a moniker that she hated all of her life.

I've known a number of individuals who decided in their teenage years, or later in their lives, that another name suited them better than what their parents originally chose for them. For some folks it's a shortened version of their given name, and for others, it's a radical departure. Angelina could prefer Angie; Jonas Arthur Harold Wilson III might prefer Bubba.

Ari's Story

One day while I was meditating, I closed my eyes and I was suddenly inside of me, *sensing* everything but not seeing or hearing it . . . just sort of *being* it. I found myself experiencing an eternal moment, where there is no time or space, it just is somehow. I began to have a vision. In my mind's eye, I "saw" my guardian angels.

The angels had come to me because a soul had chosen me as a mother! I decided to give my daughter a family name. But when she was born, and I first gazed upon her beautiful face, she "told" me that her name was "Diana."

Names are extremely important, of course, because they precede an individual into the world and create what can be a lasting first impression. Imagine that you just got a new job and learned that your boss's name was Tootsie—or Pickles? Or, say that you heard your husband's new secretary was named Tempest, Daisy Mae, or Bubbles? How would a guy in his teens react if someone wanted to fix him up with an Olive, Hortense, or Bertha? What if you found out that your new personal trainer at the gym was a woman named Pansy or a guy named Brutus?

We've all known people with unusual or distinctive names—that they themselves selected before birth, or were selected for them by their well-meaning parents. I went to high school with a pretty girl who was named Merry Christmas, and I had advertising clients named Ginger Ale, Genghis Kahn, and Chuck Roast.

And did you know that the actor John Wayne's real first name was Marion?

Brenda's Story

The first time my daughter got pregnant she wanted to name her son Hunter. But she struggled with a middle name. One day, out of the blue, I told her that she should consider the name Isiah. She was not crazy about that name, so I just let it go. But then something remarkable happened. The unusual name Isiah began appearing everywhere: TV shows, in magazines, on the radio, and even at stores. My daughter and I could not go anywhere or do anything without hearing or seeing that name multiple times a day. She finally became convinced that her unborn child's middle name should be Isiah. Once that decision was made, the messages stopped and we no longer saw or heard anything related to that name.

When baby names start to float through your mind, you are likely to be receiving direct communication from your unborn child.

Tara's Story

In 1987, I told my fiancé that when we had a son, that we were going to name him Tristan, and that his nickname would be Tristie. I knew this because the spirit of a little boy was already regularly appearing to me in my dreams, and I just knew that he was going to be my son someday.

Long before I got pregnant, I started to have visions of another child—a girl with a cap of rich black hair and huge dark eyes to match. She was wearing purple slacks with a matching sweater, and was playing in a crib. At the time, I didn't know why I was having that vision because I didn't see myself with a girl.

After we were married and I got pregnant with my first child, we were delighted to discover that I was carrying . . . a girl! So my vision of a daughter had been correct after all. We decided to call her Leah.

I was thrilled when my mother and some of her teaching colleagues gave me a baby shower a short time before Leah was born. When it came time to open my gifts, I was surprised to find a pair of boyish-looking sleepers. I went out on a limb and announced to everybody that I would be saving those particular clothes for Tristie when he came. I got a lot of raised eyebrows!

One day when my daughter Leah was one year old, it suddenly occurred to me that she was actually playing in the same crib, in the very same clothes, and wore the exact hair style as the little girl in my vision. I was so thunderstruck, I took a picture of her in that pose.

A few years later, when my daughter was three, she came to me and said, "Mama, I think I need to have a brother now." I was shocked later on to discover that Leah's announcement came the very same day that I conceived my son. The "brother" she was referring to had already been visiting with me in spirit for almost fifteen years. When Tristan was born, he looked exactly the way he had presented himself to me in my dreams.

If the name your unborn baby wants is completely different than what you were planning—rest assured that the name your baby chooses *will* probably be different from the name that most appeals to you. When I was pregnant with my daughter, I spoke to her about the names Alexandra, Jacqueline, Madison, Brett, Eleanor, and Grace. I also fell in love with the name Campbell, after I saw the CNN reporter Campbell Brown on the evening news one night. I thought she was lovely and articulate, and her name sounded very strong and classy, which appealed to me.

A few days later, my Mom called me and declared, "I have the name for your daughter! It's *Megan!*" I must admit that I wasn't initially crazy about the name. I thought it sounded too sweet and ingénue-ish; what if she wanted to start her own business one day, I thought—how powerful would that name sound? My Mom was so enthusiastic that I didn't want to hurt her feelings, so I appeased her by saying, "Well . . . that's an idea!"

The following weekend, when I was in the video store looking for a movie, my unborn daughter recommended that I rent *Father of the Bride, Part II*, with Steve Martin and Diane Keaton. It was sentimental, romantic, funny, and I loved it! Toward the end of the film, when the young doctor was introduced, whose name was Megan, I gasped in surprise. In the scene in which Dr. Megan proceeded to deliver both of the babies, I sobbed! Then, in the next scene, Steve Martin and Diane Keaton named their daughter

Megan, after the doctor who delivered her. So I got the picture loud and clear.

When our daughter was born, we named her Megan McKenna. Now, of course, it is my very favorite girl's name. And as an interesting side note: Megan, who is now a "big girl" of seven, tells me that she's going to be a doctor when she grows up—just like the character in the film.

I always had particular names in mind if and when I was ever lucky enough to have a child. But both of my babies rejected the names I liked, and at first, I was really disappointed! However, they reminded me that the choice of a name was theirs alone; after all, they argued, "am I not the one who is going to carry the name throughout my earthly life? You got to pick *your* name!" And of course, they were right. Both of my children really look like their names, and I couldn't have picked better than they did.

Winnie's Story

I was born into a family with Irish roots. I had no experience with Russia and yet, while pregnant with my second child, Russian names kept popping into my head. When my daughter was born, we named her Sasha. In high school and college she studied Russian. Now she is getting married and her future father-in-law was born in Russia.

Some souls enjoy sharing a name with many other fellow travelers on the earthly plane, like my daughter, Megan, while other souls choose names that are unique and distinctive. I remember that when I was pregnant with my son he kept telling me that he was considering the name William. When I was almost ready to deliver, he finally made the decision about his name, and I called my Mom right away. She was aghast. "*Flynn?* What kind of name is *that*? It's a last name! You can't saddle your child with such a ridiculous name! The other kids will make fun of him! Who's ever heard of a boy named *Flynn*? What happened to *William*?" When he was born, she took one look at his little face and said with a beaming smile, "He *does* look like a Flynn!" And now she talks about how much she loves the name. Don't let well-meaning family and friends try to dissuade you from a name for your little one. Your baby knows what will best suit him or her.

Judy's Story

When I was in my early twenties, I had an intuitive awareness that I would have a son and his name would be Danny—although I was not even married at the time.

After I got married, and then became pregnant, I discussed baby names with my husband, Ray. His heritage was Irish and he happily agreed to name the child Danny, if a boy; however, my stepdaughter, Amy, really liked the name Adam.

When the baby was delivered, and the doctor shouted out that it was a boy. When they brought the baby to me, I asked everyone in the room if they thought he was a Danny or an Adam. Everyone was adamant that he was a Danny, so he was named Daniel Adam.

SINGLETON OR PART OF A MULTIPLE BIRTH

Multiples are such an amazing blessing! Did you know that one out of every eighty pregnancies results in a set of twins? And if you are over thirty-five, your chance of naturally conceiving multiples increases significantly.

One of my female clients told me that when she was a little girl, there were eight children in her family . . . all under the age of six. When I furrowed my brow in confusion, she explained that her mother had four pregnancies and had given birth to four sets of twins . . . with no fertility medication or treatments!

When you first meet someone and there is an immediate bonding—a closeness—as if the familiarity had already somehow been established, it is likely that you've just encountered a twin from a prior life.

As souls plan to return to the earthly plane, they have the choice of being born alone, in a single birth, or in tandem with other returning souls who have chosen the same birth mother and father. The decision to be part of a multiple birth is up to each individual soul. Interestingly, when I've channeled for clients before they have conceived, and their angels have told me that it was their destiny to have twins or triplets, the client typically responds, "I've always *known* that! I always thought I'd have twins!"

Perhaps one of the most famous multiple births occurred long before the advent of the fertility treatments so common today. In 1934, five identical baby girls were born to a poor farm family in Ontario, Canada. The world watched in awe as photos of the

READER/CUSTOMER CARE SURVEY

We care about your opinions! Please take a moment to fill out our online Reader Survey at **http://survey.hcibooks.com**.

As a **"THANK YOU"** you will receive a **VALUABLE INSTANT COUPON** towards future book purchases

as well as a **SPECIAL GIFT** available only online! Or, you may mail this card back to us.

(PLEASE PRINT IN ALL CAPS)

First Name _____ MI. ___ Last Name _____

Address _____ City _____

State _____ Zip _____ Email _____

1. Gender
- ☐ Female   ☐ Male

2. Age
- ☐ 8 or younger
- ☐ 9-12   ☐ 13-16
- ☐ 17-20   ☐ 21-30
- ☐ 31+

3. Did you receive this book as a gift?
- ☐ Yes   ☐ No

4. Annual Household Income
- ☐ under $25,000
- ☐ $25,000 - $34,999
- ☐ $35,000 - $49,999
- ☐ $50,000 - $74,999
- ☐ over $75,000

5. What are the ages of the children living in your house?
- ☐ 0 - 14   ☐ 15+

6. Marital Status
- ☐ Single
- ☐ Married
- ☐ Divorced
- ☐ Widowed

7. How did you find out about the book?
(please choose one)
- ☐ Recommendation
- ☐ Store Display
- ☐ Online
- ☐ Catalog/Mailing
- ☐ Interview/Review

8. Where do you usually buy books?
(please choose one)
- ☐ Bookstore
- ☐ Online
- ☐ Book Club/Mail Order
- ☐ Price Club (Sam's Club, Costco's, etc.)
- ☐ Retail Store (Target, Wal-Mart, etc.)

9. What subject do you enjoy reading about the most?
(please choose one)
- ☐ Parenting/Family
- ☐ Relationships
- ☐ Recovery/Addictions
- ☐ Health/Nutrition
- ☐ Christianity
- ☐ Spirituality/Inspiration
- ☐ Business Self-help
- ☐ Women's Issues
- ☐ Sports

10. What attracts you most to a book?
(please choose one)
- ☐ Title
- ☐ Cover Design
- ☐ Author
- ☐ Content

TAPE IN MIDDLE; DO NOT STAPLE

BUSINESS REPLY MAIL
FIRST-CLASS MAIL PERMIT NO 45 DEERFIELD BEACH, FL

POSTAGE WILL BE PAID BY ADDRESSEE

Health Communications, Inc.
3201 SW 15th Street
Deerfield Beach FL 33442-9875

FOLD HERE

Comments

Dionne quintuplets circulated all over the globe, creating an international sensation.

Consider how different your life would have been if you had chosen to arrive on the earthly plane as part of a multiple birth. If you are a multiple, how close are you to your sibling(s)? Have you experienced a telepathic awareness of what they were going through at any given time that felt like an intuitive antennae that was especially sensitive? Maybe they were having a bad day and you could somehow sense that. Or perhaps you were inexplicably flooded with intuitive information about something that was going to happen in their lives—that proved to come true.

If you are expecting multiples, this blessing was made possible because the souls involved believed that if they clung together, their upcoming earthly mission would be far more productive and successful.

PHYSICAL APPEARANCE

Your baby will also determine his eye color, hair color, skin tone, adult height, and body type. This is one reason siblings can look so different. I've seen *twins* who look nothing alike.

In my husband's family of origin, there were seven children. Six of them had dark eyes and dark hair; but one of the boys had light blue eyes and blondish hair. Think about your siblings for a moment. Do all of you share the same coloring or body type? Probably not! In some families, the females end up taller than the males, have bigger feet, and might be more athletic. My darling brother Michael and I do not remotely resemble each other, yet we came from the same pool of DNA.

When we are planning each of our earthly lifetimes, our choice of physical appearance is strictly individual, unrelated to any "norm" that has already been established by other family members who were born before us. Instead, we choose our physical characteristics based almost entirely upon the issues we have selected. For example, I understand (though not from personal experience!) that it can be difficult to have a beautiful or handsome appearance. From birth, these children may be singled out for their beauty, and because on the earthly plane so much emphasis is placed upon appearance, this can become a real challenge for an individual who was not encouraged as a child to develop inward attributes. When beauty starts to fade with age, the once-attractive individual can have a very hard time coping with the loss of what others taught them to prize so highly.

In contrast, the individual who has less appealing physical characteristics is likely to be teased by other children and is sometimes criticized by their parents, who call attention to the so-called flaws. I had a client once who described her daughter's "big nose" as "too ethnic," reassuring the child that when she got old enough, Mommy would arrange for plastic surgery to take care of "the problem." At the time, the little girl was three-years-old! I can only imagine how hurtful it was for the child to grow up and recognize that her parent felt that a perfectly healthy part of her—which everyone could readily see—was physically and emotionally unacceptable. At the time, when I channeled for the mother, we discovered that her little girl was attempting to address issues that included self-esteem, confidence, and learning how not to care what other people thought. So, indeed, the child had chosen the perfect parent to help her with those issues! The child's choice of the "big nose" was just the incentive her mother needed to provide her with the necessary adversity required to resolve those difficult issues while she was still a child. Without her mother, that little girl would not have achieved the vitally important spiritual goals that inspired her return to the earthly plane. The relationship shared by the mother and daughter was truly a spiritually synchronistic interaction.

RACIAL BACKGROUND

The racial background we choose also determines our coloring and physical characteristics. Along with gender, we shift racial backgrounds from lifetime to lifetime. Because you've already lived thousands of incarnations on earth, it's very likely that you've had numerous experiences as a member of all of the earth's peoples. Take a moment and picture yourself as Caucasian, Black, Asian, Latino, Native American, or Inuit. Your baby has also enjoyed these same wonderful opportunities.

PHYSICAL HEALTH AND LONGEVITY

Other important decisions involve the state of a soul's physical health while on the earthly plane, which includes athletic ability, energy levels, allergenic sensitivities, challenges and limitations, as well as his longevity.

If you are currently expecting, your child has already made these determinations and would be more than willing to share them with you. For instance, what if your child was going to have a dairy intolerance? If you aren't planning to breast-feed, you could offer him a soy-based formula, sidestepping problems with terrible gas pains and disruptions with his sleep patterns. What if he was going to be allergic to animal dander and you have a dog? What if he had sensitive ears and would find your TV or CD player far too loud, causing him to cry or scream in pain or fear?

Because your baby will not be able to speak for a couple of years after his arrival, one of the only ways you can quickly become aware of any special needs is to ask him *before* he is born. For example, have you considered that the baby might not care for the music that plays from the mobile over his bed? Could you drift off to sleep listening to loud music that you hated? I recently communicated with the soul of a soon-to-be-born baby who told me that he absolutely detested the mobile his pregnant mother-to-be had bought for him because it played *Twinkle, Twinkle, Little Star*. He told me that if he had to hear that inane tune played over and over for *months* as he was trying to get to sleep, he'd go stark raving mad! Surprised, the expectant mother asked what music he *would* like when he was trying to drift off—and he requested that she get a CD player and several of Billie Holliday's greatest hits! When I heard that request, I laughed, but then I mused that Ms. Holliday's soft, melodic singing *would* be soothing and relaxing. And, because he instructed his mother to get several CDs, he was not going to be subjected to repeatedly hearing the same song.

Because I was almost in my midforties when I got pregnant with Flynn, my doctor was concerned about the state of my health throughout the pregnancy. Although he never disclosed anything to me, I sensed that he was also worried about the baby's health. However, when I communicated with my unborn baby, he kept assuring me that the two of us would share vigorous good health during the pregnancy and after his birth. In spite of the fact that my well-meaning friends, family, and various healthcare providers remained anxious about the outcome, I chose to stop worrying, and only then did I really begin to enjoy my pregnancy.

Prior to his birth, Flynn did tell me that he was going to be lactose intolerant, which meant that dairy products, especially cow's milk, would cause him severe gastrointestinal distress. I was not planning to breast-feed so I was already researching nondairy products that were available. I had found a wonderful soy-based formula that my unborn baby acknowledged as a perfect choice. When I channeled with him, he declared that his tummy and intestines would tolerate it perfectly. I was satisfied that it contained the vital nutrients that would allow his infant body to thrive. But then I made a huge mistake.

About a month before my due date, my husband and I had an appointment to meet a pediatrician who had been highly recommended to us by one of our other doctors. We were ushered into his office and he began to ask questions about the upcoming birth. When the conversation touched upon how we were going to nourish the baby, I spoke up excitedly and disclosed that we had decided on soy. He looked puzzled and inquired as to why we had rejected dairy formula.

I told him that our baby was going to be lactose intolerant.

"How do you know that your baby will have dairy allergies?" the doctor frowned disapprovingly. Then, in a condescending tone, he declared, "That isn't something you can just assume."

"Oh, we're not just assuming!" I happily assured him. "The baby told us!"

The pediatrician's brow furrowed in confusion. "*What* baby?"

"Our baby!" I answered brightly, patting my huge tummy. He stared back at me for a moment with an inscrutable expression before turning to my husband. "I suggest that we start the baby on regular formula and wait at least a month. If your infant exhibits an allergic reaction, only *then* will we consider another formula. I never advocate soy unless it is absolutely necessary because it doesn't have the same nutrients as traditional products." As we left the doctor's office, I was gripped by a pang of fear. *What if the doctor was right? He is a pediatrician, after all! This is my first baby, and I know next to nothing about any of this! Could I be hurting the baby by feeding him soy? Formula is the only thing that he'll be fed for a long time . . . so it has to be the right product! I've been a professional psychic for over thirteen years, but he's a doctor . . .*

So my husband and I decided to listen to the pediatrician. Just after Flynn was born, he was fed the diary-based formula the doctor had advocated. We remained in the hospital for two nights, during which time our baby continued to consume the dairy formula. The day after Flynn was born, he began to cry and thrash every time we fed him a bottle. The dairy-based formula was already wreaking havoc with his sensitive, newborn system. Every time we fed him, he would begin to wail pitifully, angrily thrashing his legs. It took hours to get him to sleep after we fed him. This went on for ten long, exhausting days.

Finally, my husband suggested I channel with Flynn's angels to find out what was wrong. When I did, his angels quickly informed me that he was exhibiting lactose intolerance. Every bottle of that formula hit his tiny stomach like a fist, creating nausea and horrific gas pains. No wonder he was howling and unable to sleep! The angels reminded me that Flynn had shared information about this sensitivity on numerous occasions while I was pregnant, and that I opted not to listen to him.

Still afraid to think on our own, we maintained the belief that we needed the approval of the pediatrician before we made *any* decisions regarding the baby. We contacted his office and explained what was transpiring. The doctor said, "Sounds like he has a dairy intolerance. I suggest you change his formula to a soy-based product."

I was furious! Not with the doctor—not with my husband—but with myself! Intuitively, I had known better! Why hadn't I chosen to exercise some confidence in what Flynn had told me—rather than blindly follow the advice of an authority figure who wasn't aware of my son's predispositions? Why hadn't I been more assertive? Why did I shrink back from being an active decision-maker in regard to my son's health and well-being? I knew full well that my husband would have gone along with anything I had wanted for the baby. So, because of *my* choice, Flynn had spent his first two weeks on the earthly plane in utter misery.

My husband immediately went to pick up some soy formula, which we began to feed him that night. It took four days for Flynn's digestive and elimination systems to balance. Thereafter, he was an extremely happy baby, comfortably falling asleep as soon as his little tummy was full of soy formula. That gut-wrenching experience provided some very valuable lessons: I learned, *firsthand*, that it is possible to receive accurate information from the soul of an unborn baby.

I learned that just because someone is an experienced healthcare provider does not mean that they alone automatically know what's best for my baby, and as a mother, it was my responsibility to do everything I could to make life as safe, secure, loving, and comfortable as possible for my child.

I also learned not to doubt intuitive information, even if it contradicted logic. The best course of action is to *prevent* unnecessary problems by considering the advice obtained through the process of channeling.

In regard to deciding what was best for my baby, I learned the value of exploring intuitive or holistic approaches *first*, if possible, rather than considering them as Plan B.

I realized that I was entitled to be heard by my baby's pediatrician, instead of blindly tolerating a condescending, patronizing, I-know-so-much-better-than-you-do dismissive attitude.

I learned that I needed to maintain faith in my channeling ability, no matter what challenge or adversity I encountered while pregnant, or as a new mom.

I recalled the numerous private sessions I had conducted over the years for physicians who inquired about the best treatment methods for various patients. The doctors were seeking to expand and support their level of patient care by getting a unique perspective from their angels in order to make certain that their own "gut instincts" were accurate. I believe that many physicians today are discovering how they can integrate their intuitive ability, academic knowledge, and medical expertise to effectively and efficiently make diagnoses, sparing their patients from unnecessary, expensive, frightening, and painful tests and procedures.

From that time forward, I decided that I was going to be a partner in any medical decisions that concerned my child, no matter how heavy the responsibility. Flynn deliberately chose me as a mother, and I wasn't going to let him down—knowingly—ever again.

Armed with a newfound, resolute determination to believe in my intuitive instincts, my hubby and I searched for another experienced pediatrician who would share our spiritual and holistic beliefs, and who wouldn't treat us like second-class citizens. Plus, we decided that although we would agree to give our child pharmaceuticals if necessary, we preferred a noninvasive, nonchemical approach, if feasible, whenever our baby became ill.

Our angels directed us to a pediatrician who was perfect for us. In fact, I was surprised to learn that the new doctor we chose was already on his spiritual path and was excited to learn about my channeling.

My experience with the first doctor taught me some very valuable lessons that I would not have learned without his help. The second doctor validated the channeling process every step of the way. When Flynn, and later, our daughter, Megan, would visit his office with a health concern, the doctor would examine them, while at the same time ask Britt and me, "So, as parents, what are you sensing about what this might be?" When I would share what their angels had told me, he would listen carefully, taking into account all of the insight from spirits. When I thanked my angels for leading us to him, they responded, "We directed you to the first doctor to help you work through a series of issues involving faith in your own instincts. That is what your child deserves. Once you rose to the occasion, you had *earned* the opportunity to work with your current physician. You might not have fully appreciated him otherwise."

When you interview prospective pediatricians, ask them about their sensibilities. You'll quickly discover how they think, what their beliefs are, and if your philosophies would mesh well. *You are the parent.* In the final analysis, it is my belief that the decisions made about your little one are primarily *your* responsibility. You are fully capable! Trust in the fact that if you weren't up to the task, your child would have never have chosen you as a mother.

TIMING

We've all heard the story about someone being honored for a particular achievement, and they reply, "I was an overnight success . . . it only took me twenty years!"

As your unborn baby finalizes his plans to return to the earthly plane, he must deliberate about the *timing* in which he will accomplish his goals, fulfill his spiritual contracts with others, conduct his healing from traumas sustained in past lives, and experience the triumphs and adversity that will help him evolve. All souls plan timing differently, according to the issues they will attempt to address and the times that other returning souls will be available to them for relationships.

What's more, a soul may choose a mother who does not expect or even *want* to become pregnant. First of all, a woman may simply not be in touch with the destiny she has planned for herself and the timing in which certain things are preordained to occur. Destiny and timing dictate whether a woman will have sex *one time* and get pregnant, while another woman can try repeatedly for several years without success.

Magdelena's Story

Christena was my first pregnancy, when I was twenty-four years old. Everything was so incredibly cosmic, right from the beginning. After the impromptu sexual experience that was to lead to the pregnancy, I sat in stunned silence for hours. The phone rang, which caused me to realize that I hadn't moved from my sofa. I literally became immobilized by the conception after it first happened. I knew, during the act, that I was conceiving. I never had that kind of thought before during sex. I was being notified by my unborn daughter, "I'm here! I've landed!" Good thing, because I was alone and completely unprepared for a pregnancy.

During my pregnancy with Christena, I moved nine times, in and out of the United States and Canada. I had never traveled so much. I made my first visit to Northern California and met a very nice woman, who took me to see a midwife in the foothills of the Sierra Nevada Mountains. The midwife lived in a remote area simply referred to as the Ridge. She was the first person to give me confidence that I really would make a decent mom. It was a significant meeting, and even though I never saw her again, I am truly grateful for her encouragement. My daughter, who is now twenty-nine years old and an avid traveler like me, has settled with her boyfriend in the most unlikely of places . . . on the very Ridge where I met the midwife!

When I was pregnant with Christena, I attended the local art school in my area and took up pottery and ceramics classes. I wasn't very interested in it or good at it, but I felt truly drawn to it. I realized much later that it had been Christena, starting to show me one of the things that she was going to do on the earthly plane. She is now a professional ceramicist, with a successful business of her own, and a clay teacher who works with little children to help them foster their creative talents. That was definitely her—not me—who wanted to take those classes so long ago.

With my second child, Jake, I rode in a camper with my ex-husband when I was eight months pregnant. It was such a ridiculously difficult thing to do, but my ex insisted that I accompany him to a summer of workshops and seminars in New York City. We stayed in a big, beautiful, old-fashioned clapboard house in upstate New York. I thought that the baby was a boy, and in those days, there were no medical tests that could define an unborn baby's gender. We had no way of knowing ahead of time. But when the mailman at the estate where we were staying heard there was a pregnant woman giving birth there, he announced that it was a boy and went out and bought the largest blue ribbon I had ever seen and tied it to the mailbox in celebration. I took it as a good omen. The home birth went quickly, and sure enough . . . I delivered a strong, healthy baby boy!

In private sessions, I've heard angels frequently point out that some individuals prevail upon their destined earthly paths with awareness, grace, and dignity—while others continually resist important learning experiences only to feel as if some invisible cosmic force has grabbed them in a headlock and is dragging them kicking and screaming throughout the entire earthly journey.

The key is to learn as much as you can about your destiny through communicating with your unborn baby and guardian angels. The communication process is exactly the same, no matter who you are speaking with *in spirit*, whether it's your unborn baby, guardian angels, or departed loved ones. Once you discover your destiny and the timing in which future events are supposed to occur, you will be virtually eliminating the rug-being-yanked-out-from-under-you sensation that occurs when one feels that they're continually at the mercy of outside influences rather than at the helm of their own ship.

In regard to life's work: this is the number one question I am asked in private channeling sessions, and I believe if more folks were aware of their life's work and could muster the gumption to achieve it, there would be a lot more happiness and contentment on the earthly plane.

Like many of the rest of us, when your child becomes an adult, he is likely to explore a number of careers before he develops the awareness of the true nature of his life's work. As a parent, you could simplify the process by asking your unborn baby now, if you are already expecting, about what he has planned. Then, in the years to come, if he develops spiritual amnesia and is clueless about what he should do, you could plant a seed by *briefly* sharing what he told you before he was born.

Keep in mind, however, that most of us do not appreciate being pushed or prodded, especially by our parents. I have some clients who are psychics, channels, mediums and other intuitive professionals who have relayed to their children what they *know* to be their life's work, and the children are resisting it because the parent was a tad overzealous when discussing it as they were growing up. In private sessions, I've had people say to me, "I'm *not* going to be a doctor (lawyer, CPA, artist, etc.,) because that's all my Mom (or Dad) talked about! I don't care if they are intuitive, I'm sick of hearing about it!" Plant the seed a few times and then let it go. Most people like the idea of figuring things out for themselves. If you subtly plant a seed, your child may think it was all his idea in the first place.

In regard to issues: if a soul has chosen to work through the issue of procrastination, he will plan for life to come at him quickly so that he has ongoing spiritual nudges to force him out of his natural complacency. If a soul is working through the issue of patience, he will plan the events of his life to move at a slower pace to help him learn to refrain from his natural tendency of creating a life that is overcommitted, chaotic, and scattered.

Remember, too, that soon after he is born, your baby may have chosen to embark on whatever healing he deemed necessary from past-life incarnations, so he will experience sporadic dreams resulting in night terrors from the time he is born, possibly lasting throughout his childhood. Whether you remember them or not, it is very likely that you had your own night terrors, too. Try not to lose sight of the fact that these dreams are very productive because they help your baby let go of hurt, loss, anger, guilt, confusion, shame, and feelings of inadequacy that may linger inside his heart and soul. These toxic pockets of residual emotion are released during sleep in dreams that replay a scenario or event from a prior life. Perhaps he had been a sheriff in the American Old West who had been gunned down by an outlaw—who was his brother! An event like that would require extensive healing. The results of these dreams are magical. Pockets of toxic emotion are released, leaving the soul with only the most positive aspects of what was learned from the experience.

In regard to spiritual contracts: from the moment your baby is born, he will begin to encounter individuals—including *you*, of course—with whom he shares spiritual contracts. Ask him now, before he is born, how you can support those upcoming relationships for his best benefit. Throughout his life, he has planned to encounter others who will teach him by example *what to do*, while others will demonstrate what *not to do* through words and by their behavior. We all need that balance to learn and grow.

Interestingly, if your baby's future spouse will not be returning to the earthly plane at the same time as your little one, then your child might marry late in life. Or, if a soul mate is returning to earth at the same time frame, your child could meet his or her future spouse in grade school and eventually become childhood sweethearts.

In addition, if your unborn baby has already agreed to parent other souls who are not planning to return to earth for many years, she may wait to start a family until she is in her thirties— or even forties, as I did!

If you are not yet pregnant, your child is still in the planning stages of making all of these spectacular decisions.

So *when* does a soul choose its mother? Souls "queue" up pretty quickly around the mother of their choice. I don't mean to compare reincarnation to the first day of an after-the-holidays clearance sale, but it's true that souls get very excited about returning to earth to evolve. The all-important choice of a mother is considered a key decision, so certain women have quite a large group of souls waiting to be born to them. This does not mean that every soul that queues up has the opportunity to return to earth in the first family of his choice. Each soul understands that they might be waiting in vain. It's a little like a cosmic standby system.

For instance, a woman might suddenly decide that she doesn't want to have children, or that her family is complete after only one baby, despite the fact that it was her destiny to have five offspring. The souls waiting patiently to be born to her would then have to withdraw and select another birth mother and father. This happens all the time on the heavenly plane.

Recently, I channeled for a woman who was destined to have three children, yet she had numerous souls queuing. When I revealed that "there are twelve souls waiting to come to you," she gasped and nearly fell off her chair! Her destiny was to have three children, she argued, so why had so many souls gotten in line behind the first three when their chances of being born to her were very slim?

I explained that this phenomenon frequently occurs because unborn babies recognize that the souls lined up in front of them may change their plans about returning to the earthly plane.

For instance, a soul may suddenly decide that he's really not ready to return to the earthly plane, even after having made all of his plans and queuing up for a certain birth mother. Then he withdraws, giving up his position to the second soul in the queue.

What's more, souls will often jockey for position. If the first soul who was waiting to be born suddenly decides that he is not ready to come back to the earthly plane, then the second soul moves up to first place. But say that soul number two did not plan to be the oldest child in the family and wanted to be a middle child? And, say that soul number three wanted to be the "baby" of the family? That would allow the fourth soul in the queue to move up to the front of the line and become the firstborn.

In a second scenario, let's say that the first three children in a queue were all keen to come together as siblings. If one of them decided that he was not ready to come back to earth, then all three would have to withdraw. Those three souls could wait to come back to that same birth mother sometime in the future, but that would be doubtful unless the woman was planning on a very large family. More likely, those three souls would regroup and look for yet another birth mother and father who would provide similar spiritual opportunities. So, suddenly, souls four, five, and six would find themselves moving to the front of the line.

In a third scenario, soul number two could convincingly negotiate with soul number one to trade places in the birth order to allow him to come first.

Or, say that you channeled with one of your unborn babies and you found out that you were going to have two pregnancies. But then you discovered that there were five souls waiting in line, all firmly convinced they were going to be born to you. How could that be possible—if you were only going to have *two* pregnancies? You could have a set of twins, and then—triplets! Do you recall the story from earlier in this chapter about the woman who had four pregnancies that resulted in four sets of twins?

Here on earth, I have friends who discuss returning for their next lifetime, and they are already voicing their desire to be born to a certain mother. I have other friends who have problematic relationships with their mothers and they are promising themselves that they will *never* make that same choice again! I don't believe in waiting until the last minute to do *anything*; but, to me, making plans for a future earthly lifetime while still living this one is a bit like discussing what you're going to have for dinner—when you've just begun to eat lunch.

Some souls like to plan many future incarnations all at one time. Do you realize that you could already have orchestrated the destiny for your next five earthly lifetimes—*before you were even reborn* in your current incarnation? In that case, you have already chosen the identity of the women who will be your future birth mothers. These women may be currently residing on the earthly plane with you right now or may be currently living in heaven watching over you as guardian angels. In fact, you could have planned to become the future child of the baby you are destined to give birth to in this lifetime. Divine synchronicity! If you're curious about this, simply ask your unborn baby or your guardian angels. A woman who is planning a family *has* to communicate with her unborn child just to keep up with everything that's taking place behind the scenes!

If you are currently expecting, your baby has already made all of these pivotal choices and is now waiting to be born with great anticipation. Wouldn't you *love* to know everything your baby has planned for his upcoming lifetime with you? The next chapter explains the criteria a soul looks for in the perfect mother.

FOUR

WHY YOU ARE THE PERFECT MOTHER FOR YOUR BABY

Chapter Profile: Now that you understand the theory of reincarnation, I'm going to share the reasons why an unborn baby chooses a particular mother; and, you'll discover the steps you can take—once your precious baby is born—to fulfill his trust in your ability to spiritually and emotionally nurture him.

Do you realize that your baby specifically chose *you* as a mother, although he had millions of other women to choose from on the earthly plane? It was vitally important for him to be with *you.* The souls of unborn children have the opportunity to choose a birth mother and father, and a second set of parents if they plan to be adopted. Souls returning to the earthly plane can also choose a single individual as a parent if they need a lot of one-on-one spiritual and emotional time with that individual to best promote their enlightenment and maturity. Your unborn baby is privy to the destiny you have chosen; he knows if you are destined to get pregnant while inside—or outside—of a committed relationship.

Recently, I channeled for a single, forty-six-year-old woman who had a nineteen-month-old adopted daughter. Her angels told her that she was going to get pregnant the following year, as soon as she met her Mr. Wonderful. My client happily shared that she had always *known* that she was going to give birth and that she would have no trouble with fertility—in spite of the fact that she was well into her forties. Then, as if to confirm the information, her unborn son began to talk with us and declared that being with this particular mother was so vitally important to him that he'd been patiently hovering around her for more than twenty-five years. As a channel, I've had souls tell me that they had waited for *hundreds of years* for a particular birth mother!

In my experience as a channel, I was fascinated to learn that the identity of an unborn baby can shift and change according to the man she chooses as the biological father. Unborn souls gravitate to the individuals from whom they can learn, and for whom they can teach. Therefore, if a client asks about a particular man she is dating, we'd receive information about the identities of the unborn babies who would be attracted to that union. If she should break up that relationship and meet someone new, then she would likely attract a new set of unborn souls eager to come into *that* relationship—*if* the father is an important dynamic. But if an unborn baby is really keen on being with *you*, and feels that having you as a mother is the most important dynamic, then the choice of biological father will not matter as much.

Therefore, a soul can begin to hover around a birth mother long before she meets the birth father. Female clients will frequently tell me that they experience ongoing dreams in which they interact with the soul of their future child. For many women, these messages provide an inner *knowingness* that a child is destined to be born—and at the same time, it also confirms the arrival of a romantic soul mate. These lucid dreams allow a woman to begin a bonding that is physical, mental, emotional, and spiritual in nature. The tangible dreams about their future children typically continue throughout the period in which they first meet Mr. Wonderful, fall in love, get married, conceive, and give birth.

If you are a first-time mother, and even if your pregnancy was unplanned, your unborn baby *knows* that you'll be up to the task because of his experiences with you in prior lifetimes. If you've been his parent in past incarnations on the earthly plane, you have already demonstrated your ability to grasp the extent of his gifts, talents, and abilities to lovingly nurture him toward accomplishing all of his spiritual agenda. You and your baby have enjoyed multiple past lives on the earthly plane, and this spiritual history forms an invisible—yet resilient and unbreakable—tether between you. Your babies gravitate to you in lifetime after lifetime, so rest assured that you have been with your little darling many times before. It is because you have so beautifully risen to the occasion for him *before* in past lives that he has so much conviction in you *now*!

Your baby already trusts that you will be the best teacher, mentor, and facilitator for him because he can recognize all of your wisdom, enlightenment, and maturity. He can see the radiant inner light that shines from within your soul and forms the tether which connects the two of you. This soul tether connects you to each of the children you have parented in all of your prior earthly lifetimes. Therefore, when unborn babies are searching for the perfect mother, they will look for the soul tether that already exists and use it as a homing device to find you.

The soul is positioned directly behind your heart in your physical body; this allows it to filter valuable information through your emotional feelings. Therefore, your emotional feelings conduct your soul's energy and awareness. This means that when you have an important decision to make and you feel an inner conflict, you would be best served by listening to what your emotional feelings are telling you to do—rather than heeding the course of action dictated by your brain. It is only through your heart and your emotional feelings that you can access all of the brilliant information contained within your soul. In addition, an individual may manifest what he most desires by examining his emotional feelings and maintaining an intense and unwavering *emotional*—rather than *mental*—passion for what he is trying to create.

Your soul is a kind of supercomputer that has unlimited storage capacity. All of the dynamics of your current destiny are stored within it. Simply stated, your emotional wants and needs reflect what your destiny holds in store. All of the intricate details about each of your past lives are also stored there. Everything you accomplished, and all of the other souls with whom you've interacted, are recorded within its memory. When an individual wants to look into her prior incarnations through the process of hypnosis, she is utilizing a facilitator, or hypnotherapist, to allow her access to the "files" stored inside her soul's memory bank. That is one of the reasons that age regression hypnotherapy, also known as past-life regression, is so safe. You are simply taking a peek inside your own soul.

Were you aware there are two different types of light that radiate around every human being? The first is an aura, which is a subtle electrical energy field that is colored by our emotions, characteristics, and habits. Some people can actually see auras, and this is a skill that can be learned. An aura is the subtle light that surrounds all living things—even trees! People who can see auras can gain some insight into the personality traits of others. If you're curious about becoming sensitive to auras, the key is to relax your mind. Then, quite simply, unfocus your eyes while staring at someone and you may begin to see the colored aura that surrounds them. A movie theater is the perfect place to practice seeing auras. Choose a seat in the back and watch people as they come into the theater. Try to unfocus your eyes and stare at the area surrounding their head, neck, and shoulders until you begin to see color emanating from that part of their body. Remember, this takes practice—but it is a fun exercise! You'll begin to discover that each individual has a different size energy field and varying degrees of color. It is also interesting to note that this same technique works if you want to see the auras of nature. For example, if you stare at the top of a tree, you may begin to see its aura.

However, unlike your colorful aura that may be seen by other human beings, soul light—which is the second type of light that radiates from you—is apparent only to *spiritual beings* like your unborn baby. In fact, all of the spiritual beings who live in heaven, including your guardian angels and departed loved ones, can observe how much your soul is progressing by observing the intensity of the light that shines from you.

Your soul light is made up of your unique spiritual attributes and intentions. These include the kindnesses you have shown others in all of your earthly lives; how you honor your spiritual contracts; how you attempt to regard others with lack of judgment; how steadily you work toward achieving your spiritual agenda to contribute to the lives of others; as well as all of the gifts, talents, and abilities you have developed in all of your prior lives, whether you are aware of them or not. In essence, your soul light objectively reflects who you are spiritually. As you continue to build your wisdom, enlightenment, and maturity, the light that shines from you grows more luminous and more incandescent.

It is this light that will provide the steadfast beacon through which your baby will be safely guided into your loving arms at birth. Once he is born, your baby will bask in the warmth of your soul light by clinging to you as he grows and develops. Your light will continue to guide him throughout his childhood, providing the vital nurturing and inspiration he needs to accomplish everything he has planned for his lifetime.

The light from your soul light will illuminate your baby's path until he learns enough about his own light to become an independent, self-reliant human being. Therefore, the more you lavish your soul energy upon your child through your emotional feelings, the more of an awareness you will create inside of him about his own special light that radiates *his* spiritual identity.

How can you share your soul light with your baby, even *before* he is born? Simply by opening your heart to him. You can accomplish that by beginning the two way communication *now*. Get in the habit of telling him how happy you are that he has chosen you as a parent. Let him know that you can't wait until he arrives. Assure him that you will do everything possible to help him achieve all that he desires. Promise that you will always be there for him. Ask him about the spiritual agenda he has chosen and ask yourself how you might support his efforts. Talk to him throughout the day; after all, once you become pregnant, you'll have the privilege of taking the baby everywhere you go.

Judy's Story

When I was still attending college, I was in a small French class and was supposed to repeat a phrase in French about being hungry. Instead, I accidentally said something in French about being pregnant! The teacher was shocked and explained my mistake in English, and the whole class laughed, along with me. Three months later I found out that I was pregnant when I was attending that French class. The daughter I gave birth to about six months later graduated from the same college . . . with a degree in French.

If your unborn baby can communicate with you telepathically, then can he also read your thoughts, like when you have a spiritually unattractive moment? How does that make him feel? Emotional meltdowns can be easily triggered by the hormonal Olympics raging inside of you. More than anyone else, your unborn child is witness to the full spectrum of what you're experiencing every day—whether it's morning sickness, gas that would disgust a teamster, leg cramps, the desperate need to find a bathroom every ten minutes, blooming acne, weird food cravings, weight gain that would impress a Sumo wrestler, and breasts that are morphing into the eighth and ninth wonders of the world.

For a brief moment, you might have some fleeting, teary-eyed, spiritually unattractive thoughts, when you wonder why you allowed yourself to get pregnant in the first place. Or how you're ever going to be able to return to work and focus on the job after the baby comes. Or, as you glance at your dead plants, whether you're actually capable of caring for a baby. Or if you can really afford a child right now. Perhaps you've been fantasizing about aliens abducting family and friends before they can give you any more unsolicited advice. And maybe you could offer your husband to the aliens, too, before he makes any more comments about how hard the pregnancy is on *him*! You might have moments when you're wondering how an ex-boyfriend is doing, and if you should Google him. Or you're thinking of ways to manipulate your doctor to schedule a caesarean because you fear labor and delivery. Or you're wondering whether you'll ever have the remotest chance of squeezing back into your skinniest jeans and looking young and cute again . . . all the while you're furiously munching on a three pound bag of Tootsie Rolls.

In my experience as a channel, I've learned that unborn babies *can* read all of your thoughts, and yet they fully understand that at times you need to vent, or are simply crying out for support, acknowledgment, and understanding. Plus, you may feel completely overwhelmed and exhausted, especially if you're caring for young children during your pregnancy or if you're still working outside the home in your last trimester, as I did.

Your baby realizes full well that when he arrives on the earthly plane, *he'll* be the one who's whining. Before you know it, he'll be a very active four-year-old who asks for a goodie before dinner. When you refuse, he'll suddenly declare, "I hate you! I wish you weren't my Mommy!" You'll know he doesn't mean any of those things. Blessedly, right now your baby knows how much you really value your pregnancy no matter how much you complain or how depressed you become at times.

Once he is born, you can continue to reassure him that you love him, that he is the most wonderful being on the planet, and that there is nothing he can't accomplish. From the time he is an infant, get into the habit of recognizing all of his accomplishments and milestones. You'll probably hear "Look, Mommy! Watch what I can do!" more than anything else your child ever says to you.

After Flynn was born, I received some wonderful advice from a woman who was a retired pediatric nurse. "Never, ever look at your baby without a smile," she told me. "Your baby will pick up much more from your facial expressions than you could possibly imagine."

No matter how much you try, you will not be a perfect parent. We human beings cannot be 100 percent at *anything*, unless it's acting like a nincompoop sometimes! As your baby grows into a toddler and then a "big kid," you'll have days when you feel truly inadequate as a mother. There have been a number of occasions when I've put my babies to bed and felt extremely guilty for my shortcomings. *I shouldn't have yelled when the kids didn't come the first time I called them! Maybe I shouldn't have given him the time out for shooting Grandma with his water pistol. Maybe I should have stayed in my daughter's room for another few minutes, like she pleaded, when I tucked her in for the night. I should have allowed her to wear the mismatched outfit to preschool that she picked! Why didn't I play one more game of checkers like they begged? I feel guilty that we can't afford the gymnastic lessons they want so badly! Am I spending too much time at work? Why don't I cook more often?*

I've found that second-guessing your parenting skills can make you completely neurotic. We all have flaws as parents. So, in the future, when you find yourself behaving in a spiritually unattractive way because you're frustrated, lonely, angry, impatient, overwhelmed by PMS, or just plain exhausted, get in the habit of apologizing to your child—or partner. For example, say you feel badly about raising your voice and screaming like a fishwife. Apologize right away! It will make you feel better immediately, and at the same time, demonstrate—through *example*—that you are an individual who can admit a mistake and sincerely apologize for behavior that was beneath your level of enlightenment. By setting this example, you are underscoring the importance of accountability to your child. He will learn from your good example. Think of how much easier and happier his life will be if he can admit that he made a mistake and then apologize for what he said or did.

Once your child arrives on the earthly plane and you discover your particular parenting flaws, you'll probably have moments when you wonder why the dickens little Jacob or Emma chose *you* as a mother. Remember that he or she can see you for exactly who you are from their heavenly perspective.

Your child is not choosing you for a mother because he believes you are a perfect human being but because he knows that the interaction between the two of you is just what his soul yearns for—flaws and all. He recognizes that he has flaws, too.

Once you are pregnant, you can rest assured that you've met your unborn baby's criteria as the perfect mother for him. After careful consideration, your baby has chosen you because of what you will offer him in these areas:

You Will Feed, Clothe, and Provide Shelter

Your unborn baby fully understands your ability to provide the necessities during his childhood on the earthly plane. Whether you live in the most opulent of surroundings and enjoy complete financial security, or have to work three jobs in order to pay the rent on a modest apartment, your baby believes that the lifestyle you will offer is absolutely perfect to allow him to learn, evolve, and accomplish his spiritual agenda. Your baby can also "see" your destiny, even if it remains a complete mystery to you.

Consider the life of *Harry Potter* author J. K. Rowling. When she had her first child, she was living on the British equivalent of welfare. As a result of her literary success, she is now one of the world's richest women. Her first child obviously desired to be born into those modest circumstances . . . and then experience what was sure to be a challenging, roller coaster transition into great wealth.

Rest assured that your unborn baby is fully aware of how you will be able to provide for him once he arrives on the earthly plane, and he also possesses the emotional and spiritual wherewithal to prevail in his life's choices, wherever your financial conditions take you.

You Will Help Him Work Through His Issues

Your baby fully understands the issues you have chosen for your current lifetime and he is aware of exactly how well you are dealing with them. From his vantage point in heaven, he can see which issues you have successfully resolved and which issues you have outstanding. You will be a master teacher for him in regard to the issues that you have already overcome at the time of his birth; and, just as important, you will also teach him about facing issues with grace, dignity, and tenacity as he witnesses your struggles. There are eight keys to helping him address his own issues:

1. Suggest to him that—unless an individual is a guardian angel in human form—he has arrived on the earthly plane with a series of issues to address. Help him understand that the existence of issues does not make him a flawed human being.

2. Demonstrate, by example, that issues are to be faced with courage and commitment, rather than swept under a rug or denied.

3. Gently and lovingly call attention to his issues as they emerge. They will become evident through patterns of repeated struggle, such as being overly fearful of trying new things.

4. Support his step-by-step progress, remembering that certain deep-seated issues can require—in some cases—lifetimes to overcome.

5. Resist the impulse to criticize or second-guess his choices when it comes to the way in which he resolves his issues. Do not compare him to other children, especially his siblings.

6. Resist the impulse to negatively judge the progress he is making in regard to reaching his full potential.

7. Consistently express pride in his attempts to learn and become a better person.

8. Help him overcome impatience by suggesting that working though issues is like embarking on a thousand-mile journey; it will be accomplished one step at a time.

You Will Help Him Build
Healthy Relationships With Others

Perhaps more than almost anything else, if your child is capable of developing and maintaining supportive, affectionate, respectful and loving relationships with others, it will help him establish a wonderful quality of life. Although he will have his own natural inclinations and reactions to people and events, bear in mind that your child will watch your interaction with others and mirror your behavior. Become more aware of how you respond to others in your daily life. Even when babies are first born, they are incredibly gifted receivers. This means that your little one will be extremely sensitive to the emotions of others around them. So, if you are stressed, frustrated, hurt, suspicious, or angry, your baby can pick up on that and it will dramatically affect him. While I do not believe that human beings have the capacity to remain balanced and centered every waking moment, we can certainly work toward that goal to create a more emotionally peaceful life for our children.

In addition, a child will mimic his parent's response to dysfunction—or chose to do the direct opposite! If a parent remains in an abusive relationship for an extended period of time, she or he is providing an unmistakable message that can affect a child's entire life. The child will grow up believing that enduring abuse is to be expected in a relationship; or, like me learning from my mom, the child will develop a resolute determination to resist abuse in all of its forms. Similarly, if a parent is unwilling to be accountable for what she does and says for an extended period, then she is providing her child with an unmistakable message that he too is not responsible for his words or actions. Or the child may be prompted to do the polar opposite, inspired by watching his parent struggling with that issue and decide to simplify his life by accepting responsibility for his choices. We all teach our children by example.

We can all relate to wanting our children to have the best quality of life possible. One way we can help ensure that is to teach them about respecting themselves, respecting others, respecting material belongings, and—as they grow older—to remain present in other people's lives by honoring their spiritual contracts.

Your child will depend on you to mentor his relationships as he grows and develops his independence. But keep in mind that your child will also attract necessary learning experiences to further his spiritual and emotional growth. No matter how beautiful, enlightened, talented, artistic, intelligent, enthusiastic or well-mannered your child, there will be others who just don't like him for one reason or another. It's up to you to help your child understand, with as much neutrality and objectivity as you can muster, that it's okay for him not to be liked, accepted, invited, included, or recognized by everyone he meets. If your child can grow up feeling a sense of unwavering worthiness regardless of the endorsements of others, he will be on the road to true emotional freedom and happiness.

You Will Acknowledge
His Gifts, Talents, and Abilities

As his doting mother, you will recognize your child's strengths faster and feel them more deeply than perhaps anyone else. By calling attention to his gifts and celebrating them on a regular basis, you will steadily help him build a self-worth and confidence than can help him prevail and triumph through his greatest adversities. I believe that every individual on the earthly plane needs at least one other human being who *knows*, without a shadow of a doubt, how truly magnificent they really are. When your child has a difficult day, he can seek you out to help lift his spirits—and we all need that on occasion!

If, however, you did not have a parent who recognized you as a child, and you're not sure how to show others your feelings, it's easy to learn. Begin now by simply complimenting the other people in your life. Single something out that impresses you. Perhaps it's the person's willingness to help others. Maybe it's someone who always has a smile at work, can make you laugh, or is a snappy dresser. Maybe it's the neighbor who is really quiet or grows beautiful flowers, or someone who holds a door open for you, helps you with your groceries, or offers friendly service in a restaurant.

Maybe it's your mailperson or manicurist. If someone is getting paid to do a job, they deserve recognition. Maybe you remember that a brother or sister did something really wonderful when you were a kid—call them *today* and acknowledge it. Start to focus on other people's positive traits, both past and present.

Then simply mention it casually as something you like and think is special. Even if it feels awkward at first, don't stop! The more you practice, the more natural it will feel. The delighted—and probably surprised—response you receive from others will make you feel joyful. Get in the habit of saying nice things to people on a daily basis. Everybody needs recognition. By the time your baby arrives, you'll be very adept at this important skill, and your precious child will be the lucky, lifelong beneficiary. In addition, by watching you, it will become second nature for him.

You Will Help Him
Heal from Past-Life Traumas

Every human being on the earthly plane has experienced trauma in his prior lifetimes. It's true that your child will embark on his healing while he sleeps, in the form of night terrors, but the majority of his healing will take place during the day when he's awake.

While he's still an infant, each time he awakens, he will find himself in the increasingly familiar surroundings of his current earthly life. That consistency is very reassuring to a soul who has just returned to the earthly plane after a previous incarnation that was filled with indescribable turmoil and suffering.

For instance, imagine that your child, in his last lifetime, had lived on the bountiful Ivory Coast of Africa in 1740. He had a loving mother and sister, and his father was a wise man in the village. While only a boy, he was kidnapped, delivered to a slave ship, made the perilous voyage across the Atlantic, and was then sold at auction as a slave. He was forcibly taken to live among strangers, whose culture was completely foreign to him, and spent the rest of his life toiling from sunup to sundown, seven days a week. He never set foot on African soil again, nor was he ever reunited with his family.

If you became aware that your child had suffered horrors like those, it would certainly help explain behaviors that would naturally result from such anguish. For instance, your child might exhibit signs of clinginess and insecurity, crying when you move out of his line of vision. Or he might need help with anger or low self-esteem. When he's a small child, he might resist your efforts to get him to do simple chores like make his bed or put away his toys . . . having spent his entire past life doing nothing but chores! And he's likely to be very protective of his friends and family, subconsciously afraid of authority figures that could—in the blink of an eye—take complete control of his life. He may be afraid of being restrained in his car seat. He is also very likely to be sensitive about his freedom to crawl, walk, and then run where he chooses . . . *when* he chooses!

In the following story, Sharon believes that she was able to heal her brother's past-life trauma—after he was reincarnated as her son!

Sharon's Story

My brother, who was five years older than me, died in the Korean War in 1956. After his death, I began to have the same type of dream every night. This dream continued—every night without fail—for the next three years.

My brother would appear in the dream *broken* in some fashion and tell me that he needed my help. He kept insisting that I could *fix* him.

On October 25, 1959, my first son was born. I never had another dream about my brother after the day my son was born. I've often thought that my son was the reincarnated soul of my brother. If that is true, my brother was right. I have been, in some part, responsible for "fixing" him. I gave him life again on the earthly plane.

As parents, we must become sensitive to the past experiences and emotional scars that are certain to affect how our babies react to the present. The best way to access information about your baby's past traumas is to simply ask him, before he is born, about which past-life experiences he is planning to heal—and resolve— in his upcoming earthly life with you. Then, after his birth, you will be armed with this awareness that can help you understand certain behaviors that could have been completely mystifying had you not known about them. As you continue to encourage and support your child, the frightening shadows of what *has been* will begin to fade little by little until he is healed.

You Will Nurture His Interests

Your unborn baby trusts that as he passes through all of the different chapters of his life, you will be emotionally available and show enthusiasm about his interests. This can be a tall order, because when he's a child, his interests are likely to be completely different from your own, and possibly change as swiftly as the weather!

Before they were born, both of my children had mentioned what their likes and preferences would be. Prior to his birth, Flynn shared that he would love the color red, and that he was going to be passionate about airplanes and flight, and he would spend his life traveling around the world. I found this utterly ironic because I am absolutely terrified to fly! But, respecting his interests, I chose to put my fears aside. I became resigned to the fact that one day, he would likely decide to get a pilot's license, or at the very least, spend a lot of time flying to distant shores. So I began by decorating his nursery in primary colors—including red—and picked up some small airplanes to sit on the shelves of his bureau. When I was seven months pregnant, I saw this big airplane rocking horse, and I went crazy. I knew Flynn was going to love it! When I checked the price, I almost had a heart attack! Without telling my husband exactly how much it cost, I put it on layaway, and by the time I had it paid off, baby Flynn was ready to rock! Long before he was a year old, he would look up and point excitedly every time a plane flew overhead, and my husband and I would exchange knowing glances. Sure enough, he's now eight, and already talking about becoming a pilot.

Prior to our daughter Megan's birth, she told me she was going to love music that was popular in the 1920s, '30s, and '40s. Once she was born, we played children's lullabies and old standbys like *The Farmer in the Dell* and *Rock a Bye Baby*. She'd squirm and fuss until

I'd switch to swing, like Glenn Miller's *Chattanooga Choo-Choo*.

One summer afternoon when Megan was four, we happened to be in Nordstrom's department store, and there was a man dressed in a tuxedo playing a piano on the main floor. Megan was fascinated, so we approached and stood there listening for a few minutes. He winked and nodded at her as he finished the song he was playing. Then, with a big smile, he said, "Little lady, do you have a request? How about *Old McDonald's Farm?*" Megan shook her head and replied, "Can you play *They Can't Take That Away From Me?*" His eyes widened in surprise and he looked at me, wondering if he had heard correctly. "That's what she asks me to sing every night before bed," I explained. Still looking puzzled, the tuxedoed musician treated Megan to a beautiful rendition of her favorite song. She happily sang and danced along with the music, amusing the other shoppers. When the song was finished, she took my hand and looked up at me with a determined, no-nonsense expression, as if she was my thirty-year-old girlfriend. "Okay, Mommy . . . playtime is over. We have shopping to do!"

YOU WILL FOSTER HIS LIFE'S WORK

Your child is counting on the fact that, in one way or another, you will help guide him toward the path that leads to his chosen life's work. Parents always lead by example whether they realize it or not.

By profession, perhaps you are an attorney, a physician, an architect, a real estate developer, or a homemaker, and your child will be inspired by you to follow in your footsteps. Or possibly, you own a family business that you will pass down to your children.

Watching your example, your child may mimic what he sees you doing, or he may choose to do the direct opposite. When a child sees his father coming home every day demoralized from a job he hates, that child is even more likely to follow the dictates of his heart so he doesn't end up like his parent.

Benny Goodman, known as the King of Swing, became the most famous jazz musician in the world in the mid 1930s. But before that time, his rise to success was fraught with terrible, ongoing hardships that included constant money woes, spending long periods of time on the road, and the public's hesitation to embrace his groundbreaking style of music. His father, a Hungarian immigrant, had a wife and twelve children to support. The best paying job he could find was in the Chicago stockyards. Year after year, Benny spent his formative years watching his father suffer in resigned silence. In the February 8, 1956, issue of *Downbeat Magazine*, he recalled, "Pop worked in the stockyards, shoveling lard in its unrefined state. He had those boots, and he'd come home at the end of the day exhausted, stinking to high heaven, and when he walked in it made me sick. I couldn't stand it. I couldn't stand the idea of Pop every day standing in that stuff, shoveling it around." A poor, uneducated immigrant father who slaved in a dead-end job was the perfect facilitator for a son whose life's work was to create a whole new style of music. Perhaps Benny Goodman would never have persevered and become renowned around the world had he not been inspired by the fear of ending up like his father.

You Will Teach Him
to Build Decision-Making Skills

One of the greatest gifts you can give your child is a sturdy confidence in his own decision making. This will allow him to gravitate toward the choices that are best for him as quickly as possible and stay his course regardless of what he encounters along the way. Learn to listen to your child and make him feel heard. You can remind your child that *he can't be confident about something he hasn't done yet.*

Your child has chosen you as a parent because he believes that, with your guidance, you will help him avoid many of life's pitfalls, including:

- Altering his course when others don't agree with his decisions
- Second-guessing his choices when he encounters hardship or struggle
- Allowing a fear of failure to cause him to abandon his dreams
- Avoiding appropriate risks because the outcome is not guaranteed
- Adopting the habit of harshly criticizing himself
- Sabotaging his forward movement by continually needing your approval or endorsement before he does something

When you were a kid, did grown-ups ever advise you to "learn from my mistakes!" How often did you follow that advice?

Probably never! Although there is no question that it is easier and simpler to learn from someone else's errors in judgment, most human beings want to learn from their *own* mistakes. And there is no question that for a parent, allowing a child to follow through with an unfortunate choice that is certain to cause him disappointment or frustration is incredibly difficult. But how else will he learn? As you become familiar with the stages of child development, you can avoid expecting too much or too little from your child. You can encourage your child to begin making his own age-appropriate decisions when he is still very young. The key is to stand back and allow him to experience the results of his choices—whether they're positive or negative. Through this process, you will be instilling in him the courage to begin depending on his own judgment. As your child slowly develops this essential skill, he will increasingly gravitate toward making better and better choices, which will help you avoid becoming prematurely grey during his teenage years!

You Will Provide the Perfect Home Environment As He Grows

In addition to all of the other criteria we've already discussed, your unborn baby has chosen you for a parent because of your economic status, your marital status, and all of the other dynamics that will make up his future home life.

Babies are born into families of great wealth and into grinding poverty. Babies are born to single individuals and into families with two parents. Still other babies are destined to be adopted. They are born to parents who are emotionally expressive, as well as to parents who are emotionally cold and withholding. Babies are born to very young parents and to older, more mature parents. Babies are born into families in which both parents work and into families in which one parent stays at home. Babies are born into frigid climates and into tropical locales. Some babies join families with other siblings, while others choose to be an only child. And some babies chose parents who have physical challenges, such as the client of mine who was born to a deaf mother.

Interestingly, babies are also aware of the likelihood of where and when their future family will move. This means that your unborn baby can already "see" if, when, and where you might relocate! Wouldn't that be an interesting question to ask him?

Throughout the years I have had mothers-to-be disclose that they felt horrible guilt about the fact that, for whatever reason, they chose not to stay at home with their babies. They ask about what their babies will feel and if abandonment will be an issue. I fully understand their question!

When I was nine months pregnant with Flynn, my husband and I decided that it was going to be best for our family if he quit his job and became a stay-at-home dad, while I worked outside the home to support the family. Like most things, at first this was much easier in theory than in practice! After Flynn was born, and it was time for me to go back to work, I felt devastated at the thought of leaving him. What would he think of me? Would he remember who I was? Would he be much closer to my husband?

Would he love me? Would he know how much I loved him? Would he come to think of me as Mommie Dearest? My hormones were still roller-coastering the day I had to return to work. With Flynn's picture clutched in my hand, I left the house feeling like I was going off to war. I had to stop at the post office, and while I was in line, a woman in front of me saw that I was longingly gazing at a photograph.

"Is that your baby?" she asked. "Yes," I responded mournfully. "This is my first day away from him. I have to go to work. I feel so guilty!" The woman shook her head and said, "What a shame. I got to stay home with *my* baby." That was all I needed to burst into a flood of tears. I held Flynn's picture to my heart and sobbed. The other people in line looked at me in alarm, obviously thinking that I was some emotionally unstable kook, but I didn't care. As the line snaked forward and I kept looking at his picture with tears rolling down my face, I began to remember what Flynn had told me before he was born. I had asked him what he thought about the fact that I was going to be a working mom, and he had reassured me that everything would work out perfectly for our family, and that he was going to enjoy lots of time with both my husband *and* me. And he was right.

If you are going back to work after you give birth, keep in mind that your unborn baby is already well aware of that. If you are feeling guilty, I hope this is a comfort to you. Whatever your current—and future—home environment offers, it proved very desirable to your unborn baby and it's one of the reasons he chose "beautiful you" as a mom!

You Can Build Upon the Successes of Past Lives He's Shared With You

Having shared prior incarnations, as discussed in the second chapter, you already have an established history with the souls who are going to be your future children. They fully understand all of the dynamics of your current destiny in regard to what you hope to achieve, and they believe that what they have chosen as their destiny will dovetail perfectly with yours to create a simpatico relationship. Your future children already know what to expect from you as a parent because of their experiences with you in prior lifetimes. And in those prior earthly lifetimes, you may have been the child and your unborn baby the parent.

It's interesting to note that long before certain incarnations come back to the earthly plane, we have already chosen the souls with whom we're going to take the journey. This means that you could have already chosen your future parents, siblings, spouse, and even children—with their consent—for a lifetime in which you're returning to the earthly plane . . . centuries from now! With each new incarnation, we have the important opportunity to continue improving relationships with others, especially those souls who have chosen to be our children.

You Can Inspire and Motivate Him to Reach His Full Potential

Helping a child reach his full potential is not about reminding him repeatedly about everything he is on the earthly plane to accomplish. Nor is it about pushing him to do something that is meaningful to you but of little interest to him. It is important for him to know that no matter what he chooses, you will be behind him all the way.

When I was ten years old, I had a mad crush on the boy next door. He was also ten, and had already grown to an astonishing six feet, five inches. His parents paved the backyard and turned it into a basketball court for him. I remember them talking endlessly about the NBA, while my heartthrob found it impossible to muster any interest in hoops as a profession—or even as a hobby! Yet they expected him to practice every day, "having gone through all this trouble and expense for you!"

Except for some very rare individuals, most people have no idea what they want to do when they start *college* . . . much less when they are ten years old! What's more, because his parents never shifted their focus, that boy had probably abandoned basketball by the time he got to high school. Nobody likes to be pushed or prodded, and kids are especially sensitive about it. They like to come to their own conclusions about what they want to do. If you see a potential in your child, or a budding talent or natural ability, exclaim over it *once* and then let it go. If the child wants to discuss it, or take lessons, classes, or get coaching, great! If the child shows zero interest, however, then "Forget about it!" as a New York friend of mine likes to say.

YOUR CHILD WILL BE A TEACHER FOR YOU

In addition to all of the other criteria, your child has chosen you as a parent because of what *he* can teach *you*. During private channeling sessions, I've had some clients ask about the spiritual contracts they have with their children, and they were shocked to learn that their children deliberately chose them as parents—not so much because of what the parent had to teach *them*—but because of what the child could teach the parent! Remember my encounter with the pediatrician who ignored my baby messages about lactose intolerance in the last chapter? That experience taught me many lessons about trusting in the advice given to me by my future son! When your unborn baby first begins to communicate, it is very important to remain open and accepting to all of the valuable information he or she provides.

Bear in mind that each soul returning to the earthly plane wants to accomplish as much as possible. Therefore, unborn babies look for mothers with whom they've shared prior earthly lives that were mutually beneficial and spiritually productive. In other words, they shared previous lifetimes in which both the parent and child were able to fulfill their spiritual agendas—or spiritual contracts—because of how they supported and encouraged one another. You have been chosen by your unborn baby either because you are so much alike, in which case you have similar issues to address—or because your personalities and issues are opposite and therefore dovetail perfectly.

For example, one of the reasons my son, Flynn, chose me as a mother is because we are so very much alike. A major issue we both struggle with is patience, and so we draw other people to us who procrastinate. I learn more about being patient from Flynn as I attempt to support him as he struggles through that issue. By disparity, my daughter Megan and I have very different personalities and issues. She chose me as a mom to teach me about flexibility and stubbornness because she is a beautiful, independent spirit who always questions my dictates as her mom. Megan is currently teaching me about compromise, which I know I need because at times I have a tendency to act like a dictator in a banana republic!

Besides assisting you with your unresolved issues, unborn babies, newborns, and small children can inspire us with their inborn humility, courage, patience, loyalty, emotional openness, acceptance, unconditional love, joy, spontaneity, persistence, faith, and ability to live in the moment.

As a mother, you will have a profound impact on your child's entire life. Celebrate the fact that your baby has chosen you as a mother based upon the spiritual, emotional, mental, and physical opportunities for growth that you both will experience throughout your relationship.

Now that you are aware of how a spiritual contract can affect the lifelong relationship you share with your child, you can begin—now, before his birth—to understand what extraordinary insights he's planning to teach *you*.

FIVE

THE COMMUNICATION LINK

Chapter Profile: This chapter features my step-by-step technique that will allow you to open the lines of two-way, tangible communication between you and your precious little one.

When you're pregnant, it's truly a time to celebrate! You're creating a miracle inside of you. And why not celebrate the blessed event *with* the little soul who has chosen you as his mother-to-be?

YOUR BABY IS ALREADY COMMUNICATING WITH YOU

Even if you're a woman who isn't incredibly spiritual, or who has had no exposure whatsoever to anything remotely metaphysical, the process of communicating with your unborn baby is going to be as natural as breathing, sleeping, or eating good chocolate.

Don't worry about other people who suddenly think that you need intensive therapy and medication because you've gone "woo-woo." From my own experiences with psychic phenomena and channeling, I'm the first to acknowledge that if you begin to speak *out loud* in an animated conversation with a spirit no one else can see while having dinner with your mother-in-law, during doctor's appointments, at the post office, bank, or at work—it *will* cause some raised eyebrows! You can, however, learn to *silently* communicate with your unborn baby—at any time, and in any environment—without anyone else being privy to what you are doing.

BEGINNING THE BONDING PROCESS

From the moment your child chooses you as a mother, which could even be *years* before conception, his soul begins to hover around you in eager anticipation of his birth. Once the little soul of your unborn baby begins to hover, you have an unlimited opportunity to communicate with him. If you're already pregnant, your baby is probably reading over your shoulder right now! By taking the time to communicate with your child, you will be building a precious bond long before he arrives, establishing an intimacy that will make the birthing process even more magical. You have *so* much to look forward to! When your newborn baby is placed in your arms for the first time, and he looks up at you, you will already *know* him—and he will know *you*. The bond between you will already exist—a connection stronger than anything else on the earthly plane, forged little by little the whole time you were pregnant.

Dr. Schnider's Story

There is no question that people bond with their unborn babies. My son, Richard, and Jenny, my daughter-in-law, would talk to their baby through the abdominal wall, and they gave her a name well before birth. They would always refer to her as Avery Elizabeth, never just "the baby."

My daughter, Terri, is now pregnant, and she is due in January. I have no science behind it, but I've got a feeling that it's a boy. It's just a feeling, and there's no reason I can give you why I feel that way, and I don't know if I'm right . . . but I just have the feeling. But, of course, I would be happy either way.

Throughout my years in practice, a lot of my patients have had feelings. Is it spiritual? I don't know . . . it's a gut feeling. I've never quantified the validity of "feelings" scientifically. But I just had a conversation with a patient today when I was doing an ultrasound on her, and I could see that it was a little girl. The patient said, "I *knew* it was a girl! In my other pregnancies with my sons I *felt* differently." She told me that she "felt" the same as when she was pregnant with her last daughter.

FAMILY AND FRIENDS CAN SPEAK TO THE BABY

Your husband, mother, sisters, girlfriends, or any other family or friends also have the opportunity to speak with the baby, and they can use the same practice techniques, too!

As you take just a few minutes a week to practice my technique, you have the opportunity to build confidence in your ability to sense and hear what your baby is trying to communicate—not only when you make the time for a private conversation, but as you're carrying out your daily routine as well.

WHY YOUR BABY SPEAKS TO YOU

Your unborn child has many reasons to communicate with you. He may want to let you know that you're pregnant the moment conception occurs, or he may want to share the name he has chosen, the colors he favors for his room, the kind of music he likes for the mobile that hangs over his crib, whether he prefers to be breast-fed or is lactose intolerant and will require a soy-based formula, the kind of diaper/bottle/nipple he will prefer, if he is partial to his crib being placed in your bedroom or if he wants his own space, and what's more, he can even relay information about what the two of you are likely to experience during your upcoming labor and delivery. In my channeling sessions, women have even received information from their unborn babies that has helped ensure their health and safety!

One of the most unusual stories I've ever heard involves one of my girlfriends and the incredible messages she received from her unborn child. My friend and her husband, both in their late thirties, had tried to conceive for over a year. One day when my friend was feeling particularly depressed her baby-to-be spoke very plainly to her, explaining that a low sperm count was the cause of their fertility problems. The unborn baby recommended that my friend's husband disrobe and sit in front of a small fan to cool off his nether regions. The purpose of that exercise was to help boost his sperm count. Immediately thereafter, the couple was supposed to have sex.

My friend thought she had gone completely nutty to believe that her baby was actually speaking with her *and* providing medical advice about how to conceive! When she shared that amazing news with me, I submitted to her that, in my experience, there was nothing unusual about a baby trying to do everything possible to help facilitate his own birth. What's more, I had heard about this technique before from guardian angels in several of my private channeling sessions conducted for women who were struggling with fertility! My girlfriend wanted to get pregnant so badly that she convinced her husband to follow the baby's suggestion, pleading that they had nothing to lose and everything to gain. One month later, she was indeed expecting.

How the Baby Speaks to You

No matter how busy your schedule is when you're pregnant, your unborn child will have the ability to consistently communicate with you, often without you realizing it. You may be wondering, being the intelligent woman that you are, how your baby-to-be could be carrying on a conversation with you, while you remain unaware of his presence? You may be surprised to discover that the little voice *inside your head* is not simply echoing your own thoughts, as you may have logically assumed. Instead, the voice you've been hearing inside your head has at times been your unborn child engaging you in a mental, telepathic conversation that only you could hear.

Remsey's Story

I was expecting my second child, and I was having a difficult pregnancy. I went into preterm labor at thirty weeks, which was much too soon for my baby to be born. I remember being at the hospital, lying on the bed with a potassium sulfate IV in my arm to stop the contractions. I felt nauseated, frightened, and completely alone. I recall crying because I was so scared and there was no one there to comfort me.

Then I heard a little boy's voice telling me that he was okay, that he loved me, and that he wasn't ready to be born yet. I could smell him, too. It was as if his aura was surrounding me . . . and that was a huge comfort. I realized that I wasn't completely alone in the hospital—I had my son with me in every sense of the word!

The moment he was born, I instantly recognized him. Now he is a big boy of four. When he says, "I love you, momma . . . this much," and spreads his arms really wide, it is exactly the same voice I heard when I was in so much distress during the pregnancy. Just thinking about his loving communication with me in the hospital brings tears to my eyes.

WHEN THE BABY COMMUNICATES

Your baby will telepathically communicate with you all the time! He will speak to you while you are sleeping, as you go about your daily routine, and when you set aside time to speak to him in a quiet environment without outside distractions.

The opportunities to speak with your unborn child are limitless! The baby chooses to interact with you at different times of day, depending on what he has to say and how he wants to say it.

For instance, if he approaches you while you are sleeping, he can provide some wonderfully vivid images that you could "see" in your mind's eye—in the form of a dream—that wouldn't be possible for him to convey during your waking hours. In fact, many mothers-to-be have shared with me that they have been awakened by thrilling dreams throughout their pregnancy—like "Susan's Story" in the first chapter—in which their baby has unmistakably interacted with them.

On the other hand, there might be some messages that need to be shared with you during the day, while you are going about your daily routine, that would be nonsensical to reveal while you are sleeping.

As you learn more about the unique spiritual interaction you have with your child, you will become more sensitive to his presence and increasingly aware of what he is trying to communicate.

While You Are Sleeping

Your unborn child often takes the opportunity to chat with you while you are napping or when you are catching up on your precious beauty sleep. He does so because at these times your mind is at peace and you are unencumbered by outside distractions.

While you are sleeping, your child may introduce himself in a dream and telepathically initiate the bonding process. Or on other nocturnal occasions, he may provide a special glimpse into the future—in the form of a dream—so that you can "see" a vision clearly in your mind's eye.

What kinds of clairvoyant pictures might you "see" in these types of dreams? Your unborn baby can choose to show you an unlimited number of poignant images, such as what he will look like as he grows up, the kind of activities he will enjoy, the issues he is going to encounter, his special gifts, talents and abilities, how he might interact with other family members, the life's work he will perform, and even the special relationship the two of you will share.

If you want to encourage your unborn child to visit when you sleep, simply ask him. For example, you might say something like, "John, (or Baby if you haven't settled on a name or do not know the gender yet) please visit me—I would love to see you." You can telepathically make this request, or you can choose to speak out loud. Meditation is not necessary, nor do you have to do anything out of the ordinary to help this process along. Have faith that your baby is present and wishes to begin the bonding process.

You may also dream about being with your baby—as his parent—in what appears to be another time and place. If you are marginally open to the concept of reincarnation, even if you remain something of a skeptic, there will be many things that happen once your little bundle of joy arrives that won't bear up under close *logical* inspection that will really make you wonder.

For example, if you have more than one baby, you may find yourself naturally forming a closer bond with the child with whom you've shared wonderful past-life relationships as platonic soul mates.

I'm always amused when a client tells me that they often have to remind their young son or daughter, "I am the parent and you are the child—not the other way around!" This happens because we unknowingly fall back into the same patterns of relationships we've had before on the earthly plane—with the same people. Typically, a child—perhaps to a greater extent than an adult— can "recall" the nature of past-life relationships. So a child will naturally resume the routine he has experienced before. If he actually was the *parent* in a former lifetime, he may find it a challenge adjusting to the new role of being the *child* in his current incarnation. Similarly, if your current spouse had been your child in a number of prior earthly lifetimes, then you'll feel an instinctive nurturing and protectiveness, and your hubby may lean on you to handle the financial responsibilities and everything else connected with running the household—much like a parent! Likewise, if one of your parents in this life had been your sibling in a large number of past earthly lives, then he or she would probably act more like a brother or sister—or friend—than as a parent.

At times, past-life patterns remain much more tangible than we may realize. Your soul's memory bank is like an intricate computer that contains files of all of your past earthly lives. Everything you have ever done or said is contained there. Those files are always being filtered through your emotional feelings, and that is why there are times we have feelings that we simply can't account for logically, because they're emerging from the soul's memory bank. This may explain why and how you've reacted to people you've known in ways that might not have made complete sense at the time!

In Chapter Two, we talked about reincarnation and how the souls travels from heaven to the earthly plane. After your darling child is born, there will be numerous occasions when you observe what might be considered tangible evidence of reincarnation when observing your child's talents and skills. You'll wonder how your child could attempt something for the first time and demonstrate obvious ability—like he's done it before and is simply picking up where he left off. *Sure didn't come from Daddy or me,* you might say with a grin.

Related to that, my son, Flynn, got into trouble at school several years ago because he insisted on serenading his entire class with his impressive Elvis impersonation—holding a pretend microphone, with an eyebrow raised, and confidently crooning to all the little girls while treating them to his dance "moves," as he calls them. My husband and I are rather shy, so we absolutely marvel at his ability to get up in front of people and so comfortably perform; however, Flynn's teacher did not share our enthusiasm for his inborn talent that particular day!

I became curious as to how our little son was capable of performing like that without ever having heard Elvis's music or seen him on film, so I decided to ask Flynn's angels. They told me that Flynn had enjoyed many past-lives in the performing and creative arts, so entertaining others was as natural for him as breathing or sleeping. Then I understood where his natural ability came from! And no, he wasn't the King in a past-life. But to this day, my husband and I still haven't figured out how Flynn learned Elvis's songs and how to move his hips exactly like him—unless our five-year-old had a secret life we didn't know about.

As You Go About Your Daily Routine

If you're like most women, you would probably characterize your daily routine as enormously hectic and demanding. In other words, you're on the go from the moment you open your eyes until the wonderful moment you climb back into bed at night.

Unless you live a life of privilege and have all kinds of people to whom you can delegate (and with the dire exception of being forced into bed for the duration of your pregnancy), you'll have to continue to get things done as you always have, no matter how you feel physically. Business as usual! With so little time to get everything accomplished, especially if you work outside the home or care for children as a stay-at-home mom, you're compelled to juggle six hundred balls at any given moment.

So how can your precious unborn baby get through to you with everything you have going on in every waking moment? He telepathically communicates when you're going about your daily routine. I call that form of channeling "on the fly." It feels like you're talking to yourself, but in reality, you're receiving messages from your baby.

Although we all receive most of our intuitive information on the fly, I believe that when the vast majority of people get spontaneous psychic messages, they don't accept them for what they are and instead start to analyze them to death. For instance, you might be involved in a certain activity, and suddenly, something completely unexpected flashes through your mind, unrelated to what you're doing—like the image of an old friend you haven't connected with in years. You might be inclined to dismiss that fleeting image, until out of the blue, that same friend calls you the next day and you're left wondering, *Is that why she popped into my head yesterday? How did I know that?* I'm suggesting that these sudden, unexpected flashes occur to reveal intuitive, or psychic, information—and rather than dismissing or analyzing it, you may want to listen and take it to heart!

When you are pregnant and you hear something inside your head, the voice may be that of your baby. For those of you who are extra pragmatic (I happen to be pragmatic-*light*), and don't want to feel like a nincompoop by *assuming* the voice inside your head is a spirit, then simply ask. For example, you could silently inquire, "Are you my baby?" and you'll receive a prompt telepathic reply—from the baby himself. The reply may come as a rush of positive, happy, intense emotional feelings, or it can come as an actual voice that you hear inside your head: "Hi, Mommy! It's me!"

At the same time you're learning how to bond with your unborn baby, you are also developing the ability to communicate with your angels and departed loved ones. The process is exactly the same. So, as you practice your new channeling skills, simply ask your baby— and your angels and departed loved ones—to introduce themselves with a specific salutation that can allow you to differentiate between them whenever they have something to communicate.

For example, when I was pregnant I always heard my unborn babies say, "Hi, Mommy!" so of course, I knew it was them. My departed loved ones usually introduced themselves by referring to me by my unfortunate childhood nickname, "Hello, darling Kimmy!" On the other hand, when my angels spoke to me, they typically began a conversation with, "Good morning, dear one," or something to that effect. Learning to clearly discern who is speaking with you will make the channeling process so much easier. If you're having a challenge trying to figure out exactly who is telepathically communicating with you, create a different salutation for your unborn baby, guardian angels, and departed loved ones—and that should easily address any confusion!

You certainly have plenty of time each day to chat with your little munchkin. Consider the fact that you're taking the baby everywhere you go for the whole nine months you're expecting. This means that every moment you're on the fly, so is he! Because you've already developed the ability to be a brilliant multitasker, why not make the most of your time by talking to your darling baby every chance you get? By developing the habit of telepathically interacting with your baby, you are demonstrating commitment to the prenatal bonding process.

For example, you could speak to your baby while you're driving, exercising, at the computer, in the shower, doing your make-up, cooking, cleaning, doing laundry, grocery shopping, waiting in line at the bank or post office, at your desk at work, waiting to be examined by your OB/GYN, watering the plants, having lunch, getting a manicure or massage, watching TV, or just before you go to sleep at night.

When I was pregnant with my daughter, Megan, I used to talk with her the whole time I was driving to work every day. Sometimes while I was waiting at a stoplight, I would see other drivers staring at me as I talked out loud, and I guessed they naturally assumed that I was singing with the radio!

When You Set Aside Private Time to Speak With the Baby

This is the most productive and proactive method of creating a clear, unmistakable dialogue between you and your unborn child. If you're wondering what you can do to build your ability to talk with your unborn baby, this is it! By devoting no more than half an hour per week, you have the opportunity to dramatically enhance your ability to "hear" what your child is trying to communicate. Remember that as each moment ticks by, you are losing significant bonding opportunities, as well as missing out on the vital information he is trying to share.

STEP ONE—MAKE THE COMMITMENT: Choose a specific day and time to set aside each week to practice communicating with your unborn baby. Consider this ongoing commitment *written in stone.* If you allow anything to interfere (unless, of course, you have a sick child) you'll never make headway. Ironically, have you ever noticed that whenever you set a new agenda, or goal, something typically occurs to interrupt your plans? Don't allow that to happen. Stick with your commitment. You'll never have this time back again!

STEP TWO—CHOOSE A PLACE TO PRACTICE: If you don't choose to set your alarm extra early and speak with the baby first thing in the morning, then later in the day you'll need to find a place peaceful enough to allow you to hear him. This doesn't mean you have to find a locale so quiet you could hear a pin drop, but you're not going to be productive in the neighborhood coffee shop, the grocery store, the nail salon, the gym, in a noisy office, at home with children underfoot, or in any other situation where you're sure to be disturbed or distracted. Keep in mind that you're going to devote at least thirty minutes each week to this project, so if the environment you choose is outside your home, it needs to be safe and secure. It doesn't matter if you always choose different environments—in fact, practicing in different places will allow you to recognize which environments and times of day work best for you.

STEP THREE—CLEAR THE DECKS: While it's true that you can talk to your baby at any time and in any environment, for you to be able to clearly hear him *speak back to you* will require the elimination of as much peripheral noise and distraction as possible. Once you become more sensitive to communicating with your baby, you'll be fully capable of hearing him in almost any environment, no matter what's going on! For now, turn off your cell phone, TV, and radio, move away from the computer, close your office door, and if you have children, why not play a movie for them in another room, or simply wait until nap time?

STEP FOUR—OPEN THE FLOOR: Once you've decided on your quiet time and place and you've gotten yourself comfortably situated, it's time to begin. Say hello to your munchkin and ask what he'd like to talk about. Be patient. Remember, this is a new skill. Listen to what you hear inside your head and trust that it's the baby. At first, you're going to believe that you're talking to yourself, and you might become discouraged or start to feel foolish. Don't stop—persevere! Have faith that the *first thing* that pops in your mind, whether it's one word—or three paragraphs—is your answer.

Begin the dialogue, and as the days and weeks unfold, you'll develop confidence that the voice inside your head *can't be you* because you're receiving all sorts of intuitive information that actually becomes a reality. This means that at times, your unborn baby will communicate things that intellectually you couldn't have known. This is possible because your unborn baby has access to all the same information as your guardian angels. Therefore, he can share information about himself, the pregnancy, and other topics that are of interest to you, such as your career, your partner's career, finances, health, where you should move, and about family and friends. As you receive this wealth of intuitive information—actual *predictions* about events that your unborn baby believes will happen, which then really *occur*—you will have tangible evidence that you are speaking to someone outside of yourself. For instance, say your unborn baby tells you that your hubby is going to get a significant raise and promotion at work, which is totally unexpected. Or your baby could share information about a move, or perhaps warn about a big snowstorm or thunderstorm that will hit your area. When these events—or any others that he tells you about—take place, it will serve to confirm that your child is doing his part to promote the bonding between the two of you—and that he is really there!

STEP FIVE—START A JOURNAL: You'll definitely want to jot down what your baby is telling you so you'll have a record of this precious and invaluable communication. He'll not only be casually chatting with you, but also passing along important information that you might want to share with your spouse or OB/GYN. I know what you're thinking. "Oh, sure, the next time I'm in my doctor's office, I'll say, 'Dr. Smith, I talked with my unborn baby yesterday, and she told me that . . .'"

What you *could* tell your spouse or physician is that you "have a sense" that this—or that—is currently going on, or going to occur, and just smile and casually shrug. No one would think that was odd. However, when things *do* happen exactly as you predicted, you're going to have some explaining to do! You could consider mustering the courage to simply tell them that the information came directly from your unborn baby. After all, the validity of the information is rather hard to question because it proved correct! Moreover, if the information could obviously not have been guessed at or concluded through mental reasoning or logic, then the *source* of the prediction would also be hard to question!

Before I became pregnant with my first child, I had already been channeling professionally for fourteen years, so I had overcome my squeamishness about divulging psychic information to strangers. At forty-four, I was absolutely thrilled to be expecting. Although I honored and respected my doctor's extensive medical experience and expertise, I wanted to pass along anything and everything I heard from my unborn baby because I truly believed it could yield additional insight. What could it hurt, I reasoned?

So, during every prenatal appointment throughout the entire pregnancy, I relayed information about my health, the gender and health of the baby, as well as tidbits about my upcoming labor and delivery. Each time I shared intuitive messages, Dr. Schnider would look puzzled and respond, "But . . . how do you *know* that?" To which I would always answer brightly, "Because he told me!" indicating the baby growing in my ever-swelling tummy. Then my OB/GYN would raise his eyebrow and change the topic of conversation. However, as I look back, everything I shared with my wonderful doctor *did* come to pass!

There are a number of very good reasons to maintain a diary of your prenatal communication. In doing so, you'll be able to:

- Bolster confidence in your ability to channel when the information you have received becomes a reality during your pregnancy
- Broaden your awareness of the extraordinary opportunity that exists for you to initiate a bond with your child—*before* birth
- Utilize all of the ongoing intuitive information available to you, particularly at times when you feel worried, frightened, uneasy, or depressed about the pregnancy or some other facet of your life
- Provide your child—in later years—with the heartfelt, fascinating journal of your earliest communication

STEP SIX—ASK QUESTIONS: Each week, you should consider compiling a brief list of questions for your baby about anything that interests you, such as what you can expect during the rest of the pregnancy, the state of your health, the baby's health and well-being, how the labor and delivery will transpire, the reasons he's chosen you as a mother, and how you'll be helping him with his childhood issues. You can ask your baby anything you like. However, if you're having a challenge compiling your list, consider some of the prospective questions presented in Chapter Six and use that as your template.

As you practice, you'll begin to hear your baby's messages. Expect that at first, what you hear will be rather soft and faint. But as you practice, the voice you hear telepathically can become increasingly distinct and tangible—sounding exactly as if you are talking to yourself in a clear, unmistakable monologue.

STEP SEVEN—THE TECHNIQUE: Assemble a notebook and a pen, or sit in front of your computer. If you choose to use a notebook and pen for this exercise, or a laptop, make yourself comfortable in the place you have chosen to practice. I don't recommend that you lie down, however, because the chances are fairly good that you'll fall asleep! Sitting at the kitchen table, on the couch, in a comfortable chair, or at your desk at work (if you have a modicum of privacy) are all excellent choices. Take several deep breaths to get centered and balanced. Tell your baby that you are ready to begin a conversation. You may speak to him telepathically (inside your head) or out loud, whichever you prefer. Ask your first question. Listen to what immediately pops into your head. Try to refrain from second-guessing the source of the answer you receive. What you hear is communication from your little munchkin . . . *not* your brain.

Write down what you hear, whether it makes immediate sense or not. Remember, you're building special communication skills. You didn't develop any of your other learned skills immediately. If you joined a gym, it would take time to develop strength and endurance. Speaking to the baby is a similar process. The more time you invest, the better (and faster) your skills will progress. Be patient! Keep at it, and trust that your baby is there and excited to speak with you. Once you receive an answer, move to your second question. Expect that at first, the messages you receive will be brief: possibly "yes," or "no," or "soon." As you continue to practice, the communication will expand, and soon you and your baby will be enjoying long-winded conversations. If you attempt to speak with your baby and you hear absolutely nothing, it could be that you are simply too tired or impatient! In that event, simply ask another question. If the silence is still deafening, put aside your notebook and try again the next day.

STEP EIGHT—PRACTICE: Like anything else, developing your intuitive communication skills will take a little time. After just a few brief practice sessions, however, you're likely to begin developing the sensitivity to hearing what your baby is trying to communicate, which will help you build confidence in the fact that you really *are* bonding with the little soul who is so eager to become your child. I've included a number of troubleshooting techniques that I share during my channeling workshops:

If you start to pressure yourself or become self-critical, this magical process will be as much fun as cleaning out the refrigerator.

Not to belabor the point, but have you ever noticed that when you're pressured to find something to wear for a certain event, it can take all the fun out of shopping? Or if at work you're pressured to complete a project, that instead of being stimulating—it's nothing but stressful? You get the idea. Tell yourself, *I am not attached to the outcome. I will practice and my ability will develop in its own time.* Keep it fun! After all, you're endeavoring to begin the bonding process with the little soul who has gone to great lengths to deliberately choose *you* as a mother.

If you can't hear or feel the presence of your unborn baby even after you've practiced a few times.

You *can* become very adept with this skill! Channeling, the process by which you can speak with your unborn baby, is usually simpler for *feelers* than for *thinkers*. But even if you are a female Einstein, you can do this! Do you realize that your beautiful brain is where all of your negative tapes run? For instance, you'll know you're *thinking* instead of *feeling* when you sit down to talk with your baby, and instead of hearing the baby, your brain starts to tell you, *I'll never be able to do this, I'm just talking to myself. I'm probably not hearing correctly, My husband thinks I'm crazy. My baby will think I don't want to bond with her. She'll think I'm Mommie Dearest. What if she changes her mind about coming to me?*

I've found that the easiest way to quiet all the brain's negative chatter is to simply ask it to shut down. "Brain, shut down." While it's true there are more elaborate methods by which you can accomplish the same thing, I've always favored the simplest and fastest ways to get things done. If you remember to do this on a regular basis, your brain will cease to present all of that negative, demoralizing, useless rhetoric—and you'll be able to hear your baby's messages loud and clear.

Another great way to skirt the negative mental chatter is to haul yourself out of bed extra early and talk to your baby then, *before* your brain has a chance to become active and inform you that you can't do what it is that you're already doing! Your brain telling you that you can't communicate with your unborn child is the equivalent of your brain telling you that you can't breathe.

If you can hear your unborn baby at some times, but at other times it's a challenge.

You may be worrying a lot, and that causes your brain to run amok with all sorts of negative, pessimistic self-talk, completely drowning out what your baby is trying to tell you. I would compare that to sitting in a noisy club or restaurant and trying to engage in a private conversation. Or you may have waited until the end of the day when you're completely exhausted, which certainly puts a damper on your ability to access channeled information.

How can you tell if what you're hearing is coming from your brain—or your unborn baby?

First of all, remember to shut down the brain. Once you've done that and you begin to hear conversation flooding into your head, just listen. Then, *ask* if your baby is speaking with you. "Baby, is that *you*?" He or she will answer to the affirmative, and this begins the two-way communication that I refer to as *hooking in*.

You will receive messages from your unborn baby through any—or all—of these methods:

- A rush of unmistakable emotional feelings when he's present, or after you have asked him a question. For instance, say you've asked your baby a question about how close the two of you will be once he's born. If he wished to communicate to you through emotional feelings, you'd be immediately flooded with clearly identifiable feelings of joy and peace, so intense they may bring happy tears to your eyes.

- Telepathic words that you clearly hear inside your head, as if you are talking to yourself.

- A voice that you hear clearly *outside* of your head, just like when you converse with a human being. But this will be the voice of your unborn baby as he will sound in childhood, or even adulthood, in his upcoming earthly life with you. If you have other people in your life who are intuitive, they might hear it, too!

- Symbolism or pictures that you "see" in your mind's eye while awake or asleep. For example, let's say that your doctor has determined that your due date is January 14, and you decide to ask your unborn baby when he'll actually be born. Suddenly, during waking hours, you begin to see the number nine everywhere: on license plates, phone numbers, grocery store receipts, etc. Or, perhaps when you're sleeping, you'll "see" the number nine floating in space or on the page of a calendar. Therefore, you might conclude that your baby is trying to convey that he will be born on January 9!

- Music, colors, or smells that become apparent while you're awake or asleep. Let's say that your doctor has predetermined your due date to be early January. Then in your sleep you're bombarded with Christmas carols, Hanukkah songs, snippets of your favorite holiday films, visions of snow, red ornaments, blue Stars of David, or even the smell of roast turkey—your family's traditional holiday meal. Therefore, you can rest assured that your baby is coming before the end of the year!

- Conveyed by another human being through the process of channeling: this is a wonderful phenomenon that happens more often than you can imagine! Let's say that right after you've discovered you're pregnant, you ask your unborn baby to confirm his presence and share what his gender will be. Then, long *before* you begin to "show," a complete stranger approaches and says, "Congratulations on your little girl!"

As you practice, you will build a strong level of confidence that your baby really is present and providing messages to you, and that you're correctly hearing what he or she is trying to communicate. Trust in the *first thing* that pops into your head after you ask the baby a question.

Why does the current telepathic information coming from your unborn baby contradict previous messages he has given you—like the timing of something that was supposed to happen?

When you are receiving messages from your unborn baby, always keep one thing in mind. *Information that he has previously given you can change.* Why is that? Because the probability of certain situations occurring—and the timing in which they are predicted to occur—can shift on the earthly plane, regardless of its connection with something your unborn baby or guardian angels have told you. There are four variables that can cause a situation, or timing, to change.

First, you may have chosen not to do something that your unborn baby or guardian angels directed you to do. Example: say that in your first trimester, you're sitting at your desk at work, and suddenly, you feel your unborn baby around you. You receive the unmistakable message that you must hurry to a certain furniture store to buy the crib you really want because it has just gone on sale. You immediately call your husband, who suggests that you wait until later in the pregnancy to start buying baby furniture. Then you call your mother, and she recommends the same thing. What they tell you has made logical sense. So you decide to wait until later in the pregnancy. In your seventh month, you decide that it's time to go shopping for the crib. The saleslady at the baby furniture store tells you that the crib you really wanted went on clearance six months prior, and now is no longer available. The saleslady goes on to explain that all of the similar cribs are on back order from Canada and are not scheduled to arrive for four months. What's more, the cribs that are available do not appeal to you and cost twice as much as the dream-crib did on clearance. You find yourself asking, *Why didn't I listen?*

Second, situations and timing can shift because another human being failed to do something that they were directed to do by spirit. Example: your OB/GYN has recommended a caesarian. Your husband can't take an extended leave from his job, so you've asked your sister to stay for a few weeks to help with the baby after the birth. Your unborn baby and angels assure you that your sister will rise to the occasion. However, the day before the scheduled birth, your sister phones to announce that staying with you is going to be too much work for her and she's decided not to come. Her failing to rise to the occasion for you, at the last minute, is as much of a surprise to your angels and unborn child as it is to you. When another human being fails to rise to the occasion—a situation over which you have no control—your unborn baby and guardian angels will mobilize to quickly devise a Plan B that will achieve a similar objective. Have faith that you are not alone when other human beings let you down. It *will* happen from time to time.

Third, whatever you were originally told by your unborn baby or guardian angels shifted dramatically because there was something emerging behind the scene that was altogether better. Example: you are in your first trimester and really keen to buy a house with a small yard for the baby. After extensive searching, you and your hubby find a cute three bedroom house that needs some renovating, in a decent neighborhood, with good schools, and moderate taxes. You ask your unborn baby about the house, as well as your angels, and they all tell you that the house will soon be yours. However, two months later, when you are in your fifth month of pregnancy, the deal falls through right before closing. You respond by being very frustrated, angry, and depressed. You and your husband begin the home search all over again. A week later, you find a new house, with a big fenced yard, in a better school district, that's almost twice the size of the house you lost, and for less money! The builder is even willing to offer incentives like thousands of dollars for decorating or an in-ground pool. Plus, you can move in immediately. You find yourself asking, *Why did I get so upset when we lost the first house? I should have known that it was because there was something even better for us!*

Fourth, your unborn baby changed his mind about something after he provided the message to you. Example: for the first eight months of my pregnancy, our unborn son kept talking about how much he liked the name William. My husband and I began to refer to him as William. For eight long months, except when I was channeling for a client, I talked to him all day, every day, referring to him as William. Then, in my ninth month, he abruptly changed his mind and decided on the name Flynn. For about the first three months after his birth when someone would ask his name, I would reply, "William. Oh, no . . . ha ha . . . I mean . . . Flynn!" People would look at me as if I was a nincompoop, unable to remember the name of my own child. Even after you're pretty far along in the pregnancy, your baby continues to have the prerogative to change almost anything he chooses—except his gender.

Any, or all, of these dynamics can cause events, situations, or timing to change from what spirit previously indicated. For example, if you had watched a newscast last week and then tuned in today to see what was going on in the world, you would expect the news to be different *now* than it was *then*—right? So don't let this discourage you when communicating with your baby! He may have shared a piece of news last week that he now indicates has changed completely. Expect it. That's why it's so important to speak with your baby *at least* on a weekly basis—if not every day. In doing so, you will keep your ear to the ground and remain privy to the latest, most up-to-date intuitive information, in addition to proactively developing the most precious bond you will ever know on the earthly plane.

If you know other pregnant women, you can broaden your communication skills by asking them to be channeling buddies. Get together and practice by asking for messages from each other's unborn baby. Ironically, we can actually be more confident receiving information for someone other than ourselves. Try this technique! I know a number of women for whom this has been very successful. And it's always fun to have someone else channel for you.

The more you practice, the faster you're going to build your ability. Tell yourself that there is *no reason you cannot do this*. Your baby is present and eager to interact and start the bonding process. Whether you choose to respond is completely up to you. Seize the moment! There is no time like the present.

Loved Ones in Spirit May Visit With the Baby

At my seminars, I'm always amazed by how many women share their heartwarming experiences of being visited, at night while they sleep, by their soon-to-be-born baby—*accompanied* by deceased family and friends who are joyfully interacting with the child as they all wait for the upcoming birth to take place.

When my client Susan was pregnant with her first child, she lost her mother to cancer. Susan was heartbroken, not only from the loss of her mother and best friend, but also because she was convinced that her baby would never know his grandmother. More than ever before, Susan really needed her mother—and her mother would have given anything to remain with her. But fate tragically derailed their beautiful plans. At a loss with how to cope, Susan came to me for a channeling session a month before her baby was born.

When I began to channel, I "saw" Susan's mother holding her unborn child in her lap, and there were two other children standing right beside her! They were all together, happily awaiting each of the upcoming births. Because we already knew that Susan's current pregnancy was a singleton, we realized that the two other children had also chosen her as a mother. Susan's mother was able to provide all kinds of delightful, detailed information about the due date, the labor and delivery, the gender of the baby, the child's likes and dislikes, and what his life's work was going to be. She also informed Susan that she remained president of her fan club, which made Susan chuckle, and that she was still very much present, and as loving and supportive as ever. She announced that she would indeed be there every step of the way—just as if she was still on the earthly plane in a physical body.

A little over a month later when the baby was born, the birth took place exactly as her mom said it would. Susan is now pregnant with her second child. Her firstborn, who is now three, often mentions his grandmother "Mimi" and repeats conversations they have. Susan truly believes that her mother is with her in spirit form because she can tangibly feel her presence, and what's more, Mimi relays clairvoyant information that foretells circumstances and events that become reality. Susan now channels for herself and happily speaks with her mother every day.

I've also had numerous clients ask if perhaps their new baby is the reincarnated soul of a departed family member because they look so much alike or a toddler or small child exhibits the same gestures, facial expressions, or phraseology as a deceased family member. However, I've found it to be fairly rare for a loved one to choose to be born back into the same family from which he just departed.

The easiest way to ascertain whether the soul of a departed loved one has returned through a birth inside the family is to simply attempt to channel with the soul of the family member. If he "speaks" to you telepathically, then you know that his soul still resides in heaven and therefore is not housed inside a human body on the earthly plane. If you receive no telepathic response when you attempt to speak with your loved one, then you can ask one of your angels.

I know that it's extraordinary, but it is possible for two completely different individuals—one residing on earth and the other in heaven—to have the same mannerisms, patterns of speech, facial expressions, and even the same laugh. Remember that we've all shared numerous past lives on the earthly plane. It reminds me of that old adage about how much a married couple begins to resemble each other after they've been together for a long time.

After so many incarnations, we're bound to share some of the same traits!

As you practice the techniques that I've shared, you'll be able to build upon the natural psychic ability that emerges so profoundly when you are pregnant. If you're willing to explore your ability, you'll dramatically expand your awareness of your baby's presence. And if you choose, you'll be able to detect the presence of your angels and loved ones in spirit as well.

SIX

TOPICS to DISCUSS WITH YOUR BABY

Chapter Profile: As you continue to hone the skills that you've learned in Chapter Five, have you considered which new topics you'd like to discuss with your unborn baby? In this chapter you'll find a vast array of possible questions that you can ask your future child to help you get to know him and allow the all-important mother/child bonding process to fully blossom.

As you practice communicating with your unborn baby, I urge you to maintain a journal consisting of your little one's messages. The journal will help you develop an increasing confidence about the bonding process. Being receptive to the communication will also help you become the best possible parent for the special being who has gone to great lengths to become a very precious part of your life on the earthly plane. And imagine how extraordinary and unique a gift it would be to share the journal with your child when he or she is old enough to appreciate what is inside.

What's more, the information that you receive from your unborn baby can be shared with family members and close friends. I wouldn't be surprised if you contacted members of your family with a message you'd just heard from the baby—and discovered that your baby had already communicated the same thing to them!

One thing is certain: we live in a remarkable universe. Don't let another day go by without opening the lines of communication with the soul who has honored you with his or her future. Keep in mind that you can discuss anything you wish with your baby, and the questions you may pose are limitless. In addition, if destiny dictates that you will have more than one child, you may hear simultaneous messages from two or more unborn babies.

The following list of questions is meant to be a starting point from which you can build the spiritual and emotional bonding between you and your child.

QUESTIONS FOR YOUR UNBORN CHILD

Pregnancy and Birth

When will I/did I conceive?

Is there anything more I can do—for my part—to become, or stay, pregnant?

Will the pregnancy be healthy? Any foreseeable problems or challenges? If so, what can I do about them?

What will be your date of birth? Time of birth?

What will I experience in labor and delivery?

Will your birth involve a vaginal birth or a caesarean?

What can I do to make labor and delivery as pleasant as possible?

Who would you like to be present at your birth? Should we photograph or film the actual birth?

I am considering an epidural (natural childbirth, induction, home birth, water birth, etc.); what do you think of my choice?

Can you predict your birth weight? Length in inches?

What will you look like? Eye color? Hair color? Adult height/body type?

Family Bonding

Why did you choose me as a mother?

Why did you choose your birth father?

If you will have siblings, why did you choose them?

What can I teach you?

What can your father teach you?

What can other family members teach you?

What are you planning to teach me? What are you planning to teach your father? What are you planning to teach other members of the family?

Are there any family members who are your soul mates?

Have you picked out a first and middle name?

Are you planning on coming alone—or as part of a multiple birth?

If you're going to be part of a multiple, how many babies are coming with you?

Are they available for me to speak with right now?

Your Baby's Preferences

When we first bring you home, would you prefer to sleep in my room or in your own bedroom?

What would help you most easily adjust to life outside the womb? Certain types of music? Massage? Being carried in a papoose-type carrier against my body?

Once you are born, will you be frightened of anything in our home . . . like family pets, etc?

Do you like the pediatrician we have chosen?

What will be your favorite colors, music, books, and toys as an infant and baby?

As a baby, what will be your favorite places to visit? The park? The beach? Grandparent's house? The zoo, etc?

As an infant and baby, what will be your favorite type of formula/foods? Least favorite?

What kind of diapers will you prefer?

Will you have any food intolerance or allergies throughout infancy and childhood? Will you have any physical/health challenges throughout infancy and childhood?

I work outside the home, so on weekdays other adults will care for you. How will you feel about that? What can I do to make you feel safe and secure?

Your Child's Physical and Spiritual Health

What can I do to promote your greatest healthfulness?

What are the issues you have chosen? How can I assist you in resolving them? Will you have any fears or insecurities that I can help you resolve? In which past life did those fears or insecurities originate?

Am I currently struggling with any particular emotional or spiritual issues that you would like me to resolve before your birth?

Your Child's Future

What is the nature of your life's work? When do you anticipate that you will begin your life's work? What can I do to promote your awareness of your life's work?

What are your special gifts, talents, and abilities? How can I help you become aware of them?

Is it your destiny to marry? Do you plan to have children of your own someday? When?

You and Your Family's Past and Future

Do you know if any other souls are already planning to
follow you and join our family later? Girls? Boys?
Singletons or a multiple birth? Will I conceive these
children or will we adopt, use a surrogate, etc?

Can you relay information about your past lifetimes? Can
you shed light on the past lifetimes we have shared on the
earthly plane? Was I your parent in the past? What did we
accomplish? What challenges did we encounter?

Do you ever see Grandma, Aunt Vera—or any other departed
relatives or friends? Do they have any messages for me or
anyone else? Do you spend any time with my angels?

Channeling

How can I tell if it's you that I "hear," not one of my angels
or departed loved ones? What are the names of the angels
who will be working with you once you are born? Will any
of our departed loved ones be working as an angel for you?
Can I help you by communicating with your angels
myself?

ADDITIONAL QUESTIONS
IF YOU ARE EXPECTING MULTIPLES

Why did you decide to come together?

What do you expect to learn from each other?

Have you encountered one another before in prior lives?

Have you been part of a multiple birth in prior lifetimes?

Who will be born first? Why?

How will you support each other? Will you be emotionally close—or feel competitive? Will there be any telepathic interaction between you? How can I become more aware of it so I can encourage your bond?

Will you be as close to your other siblings as you are to each other?

How can I best support your spiritual agenda? How can I best support your good health? Will you share similar challenges—like the same allergies?

Will your personalities/likes/dislikes/preferences be similar— or more dissimilar? Have you chosen your names yet?

How important is it for me to distinguish you as individuals by dressing you differently, making certain you're in separate classes at school, etc?

SEVEN

INTERPRETING YOUR PREGNANCY DREAMS

Chapter Profile: When you're pregnant, you're super psychic. You're going to have more dreams than ever before, and they will be very vivid and colorful. Some of the dreams will convey beneficial intuitive messages that originate from the baby, your soul, angels, and departed loved ones. At the same time, raging hormones, fear, and exhaustion create weird nightmares that you may already be experiencing. Find out where all of these dreams originate, and discover the necessity of creating a dream journal to help you differentiate between the dreams you should completely ignore—and which dreams you must heed because they're providing important messages.

Lights! Camera! Action! Quiet on the set! Are you about to watch the filming of a new movie? No . . . you're pregnant and about to go to sleep! The dreams will begin sometime after you lay your gorgeous head on the pillow, filled with more melodrama than three daytime soap operas could possibly portray in a year.

Even if in the past you haven't remembered much about your dreams, that's about to change. At a certain point in your pregnancy—often in the first trimester—you'll suddenly become the recipient of unexpected movie-of-the-week-type nightmares. Combine raging hormones with unsettling feelings of fear, anxiety, and stress about the baby and your ability to mother, and you've got the perfect formula for generating dreams unlike anything you've ever experienced.

At the same time, you'll be experiencing fabulous *intuitive* dreams as a result of visits from your unborn baby, guardian angels, and departed loved ones who convey useful information about your present and future destiny. You'll also discover that from time to time your soul will share information about your past lifetimes that can enhance your current quality of life. Now you know why you feel so tired when you wake up some mornings! Many of these slumbering adventures are likely to continue until your darling little one is born. Whether you are settling in for the night or grabbing a catnap during the day, you'll have more vivid, dramatic dreams during your pregnancy than at any other time in your life, and they'll rival anything you'll ever see on-screen.

Let's begin by exploring the six basic elements that allow a dream to take shape:

ELEMENT ONE:
THE TWO DIFFERENT TYPES
OF PREGNANCY DREAMS

When you're pregnant, you will experience two *very* different kinds of dreams: valuable psychic/intuitive dreams, and fear-based nightmares.

The key is to learn how to differentiate between the mental fear-based nightmares—which you should simply ignore—and the valuable, comforting intuitive dreams that relay meaningful information. Initially, both types of dreams are certain to get your attention. If you were to think of these dreams in terms of your personal life, the nightmares would be comparable to meeting an immature, commitment-phobic, self-absorbed Mr. Right Now, while the meaningful intuitive dreams are similar to connecting with a Mr. Wonderful. Although we eventually encounter both types of men, being able to differentiate between them *as quickly as possible* means everything.

Psychic/Intuitive Dreams

These dreams are typically positive, comforting, or exciting, and provide you important visceral, insightful messages from your unborn baby, guardian angels, departed loved ones, and even your soul. Before you conceive and during pregnancy, your unborn baby is likely to communicate with you as frequently in your dreams as he will telepathically during your waking hours because you are a captive audience while you sleep.

Telltale sign: You awaken refreshed, happy, at peace, and *knowing* that you received contact because of what you recall having seen, heard, smelled, or touched in the dream.

Psychic or intuitive dreams may focus your attention—or provide worthwhile information—about the past, present, or future. The source of the information about the *present* and *future* is usually provided by your unborn baby, guardian angels, and departed loved ones. For example, you may have a dream in which the baby has already been born and you'll be able to see what he looks like, how it feels to cradle him in your arms, and the bliss you'll experience when your eyes meet. You may also have prophetic dreams about what you can anticipate for the rest of your pregnancy, what you'll experience in labor and delivery, and how it will feel to take the baby home. As much fun as it is to play with all of your baby clothes and toys, actually spending time with the baby—while you sleep—will be a lot more satisfying! As you interact before his birth, the bonding will begin and flourish, so when he is born, you two will already know each other.

Belin's Story

As soon as I was engaged to be married to my husband, Roger, I began to have very vivid dreams about three children who were eager to talk and be with me. One female was always in the forefront, waving her hands excitedly and eager to communicate. The other two children, who were male, were patiently making their presence known, quietly waiting in the background.

The dreams were frequent and powerful. When I'd wake up, I couldn't shake the visions. I knew that the dreams were important because I rarely remembered dreams unless they struck a deep chord within me. After talking to my mother, Rebecca, who is in tune with spirit, she confirmed what I had been feeling and knowing all along. These spirits were children waiting to be born to me. It was beautiful, and I felt honored by their excitement, but I was also a bit scared. I had not finished college, my husband had barely started college, and we felt we were just not ready on many levels.

After talking with my wise mother, she advised me to just let the spirits know that it was not the right time, and that our children would be welcomed when we were ready to start a family.

I talked with all three of my unborn babies to let them know they were wanted and loved, but that I would let them know when we were ready. I felt that the message got through because the dreams came to an end, although their presence never completely faded. They were calmly waiting, allowing us to prepare.

When my husband finally graduated college and circumstances allowed me to stay at home, we decided to start our family. As soon as we started trying, BOOM—I got pregnant! Our unborn daughter was ready . . . yesterday!

A short time after I found out I was pregnant, my appendix burst. Although I had a really rough recovery after the surgery, my daughter, Bella, fought all odds to get here. Her fighting spirit kept her alive—and that was the only kind of spirit that could have survived such an ordeal.

Now my little fireball Bella is my buddy in everything I do. Currently I'm happily pregnant with my second child, and I'm quite sure it's a boy. So what about baby number three? There were three spirits who came to me in the dreams, after all. I can feel that spirit waiting to be born, although I strongly feel like he wants to be born close to his older brother. They seem to want to come as a team, as a pair. Actually, I felt them so much in the same wavelength that I wondered if they would be twins!

The source of information that reflects the *past* typically originates from your soul. Your soul will "speak" to you during your earthly life through your emotional feelings and dreams. While you are pregnant, it escalates its communication because that magical period is a time of so much profound transition. When you're sleeping, the soul may, through a form of effortless self-hypnosis, allow you to review its memory bank of past lives that were significant for you and your baby, in which the two of you supported one another through turmoil and triumph.

Since your soul contains a record of everything you have ever experienced in all of your past lives, as well as a record of the destiny for your current life, it is a fabulous source of self-awareness. When you sleep, your soul will provide glimpses—through mental images that you "see" in your mind's eye—by projecting you back into more recent, or even ancient, earthly incarnations. Your soul offers a reflection of what you've already experienced in the past to provide a reality check in regard to challenges you're facing or a stress point that exists in your life.

For example, let's say that right now, you are fretting about your ability to properly parent your soon-so-be-born baby. That's a cue for your soul to provide you, in a dream, a bird's-eye view of a prior life in which you were a nurse in a hospital, caring for a number of babies all at the same time. That happy jaunt down memory lane would allay some of your fears, would it not? Or let's say that you are worried about how much your body will change following the pregnancy and birth, and whether your partner will continue to find you desirable. In your dreams, your soul could allow you to return to a prior life in which you shared a marriage with the same man . . . who remained steadfast and loving after you were disfigured by a case of smallpox. By returning to the past, our soul provides a brilliant reality check to help us put the *present* into a more positive, agreeable perspective.

How can you tell if a dream reflects past-life images? You'll discover that it is not difficult to make the distinction between the past, present, and future. Dreams from your unborn baby and angels usually convey information about the present or future. This will become apparent through seeing yourself and others as your current genders, wearing modern clothing, riding in modern vehicles, as well as recognizing familiar surroundings. However, in a dream that reflects a past life, you may be wearing clothing from another period, see a horse-drawn carriage or some other outmoded source of transportation, see yourself as a different gender or at another chronological age, see a person who is in your present lifetime fulfilling another role—such as learning that your current sister was your mother in the past.

In past-life dreams, you often get an exciting indication of the type of work you conducted in the past, such as "seeing" yourself as a blacksmith, the captain of a Viking ship, a cook toiling over a large cast-iron pot inside a huge hearth, a musician performing for royalty dressed in eighteenth-century attire, or a fisherman living on a Pacific island. When you "see" these images, they can inspire intense feelings of emotional familiarity—a *knowingness*—inside of you.

Rest assured that these dreams will occur at the time when they are necessary to help you resolve a certain issue, let go of fear, or take an important risk that can help move your life forward. For instance, wouldn't it be wonderful to "see" how you gave birth in a prior life to remember how you got through it before? You can, by asking your soul to reveal insight from its memory bank before you go to sleep by allowing you to witness more of your personal history through your dreams. But keep in mind that your soul will decide when and how to take you on a journey down memory lane.

Your baby's father, and even the grandmothers-to-be, can experience prophetic dreams as well.

Brenda's Story

I had a dream experience related to my grandson Hunter prior to his birth. In my dreams, I saw him as a Roman warrior standing in a horse-drawn chariot. This man was a leader and very well respected because he fought to protect those around him. He had light blond hair and sky blue eyes, and he was a very gentle and caring man who was sincerely interested in the well-being of others.

When Hunter was born, he had the same light blond hair and sky blue eyes that I had seen in my dream. When my grandson was less than a month old, he began looking off into the distance and smiling. That was not the gaze of a month-old child! You could tell there was an angelic presence around him. He has already touched so many lives in such a short span of time that I believe he is an angel himself.

Fear-Based Nightmares

These dreams are always frightening, stressful, and negative, and they are a result of mental fears or anxieties. Blessedly, these pregnancy nightmares will stop after you have the baby.

Telltale sign: You awaken feeling scared, pessimistic, worried, depressed, or confused—haunted by what you recall having seen, heard, smelled, or touched in the dream.

When I started to experience these weird, scary dreams, I thought I was going certifiably crazy. One night when I was three months pregnant, I had a graphic, detailed dream about my husband having wild sex with another woman. Although I completely trusted my husband, the dream seemed so real! And since I was a professional psychic, I woke up furious with him—certain that what I "saw" actually happened. I was so upset that I was crying, convinced that he was going to leave me. He assured me that nothing of the sort would ever take place. A short time later, I began to dream that I was in the throes of passionate lovemaking with an old boyfriend, which I had zero intention of doing, so I realized that something else was afoot. In my first trimester, I also dreamed a lot about giving birth to an adult—as if my baby was full-grown when he was born—and about tall buildings and water. As my pregnancy progressed, the dreams did too.

My pregnancy nightmares were in part triggered by my fear of not knowing what to do once my baby was born. I had never even *held* a baby before, and I had no experience whatsoever with infants or toddlers. I maintained serious doubts about my mothering skills in spite of the fact that my mom kept repeating, "Once the baby comes, you'll know exactly what to do . . . it's *nature!*"

I was resigned to the fact that I was not predestined to morph into Suzi Homemaker just because I had ovaries and had given birth. I couldn't even figure out how to make the self-cleaning feature on my oven work. Although I was a mature woman who ran a business, had written two books, and could talk to angels, the closest I had ever come to nurturing a baby was caring for my cat. So my pregnancy nightmares progressed fast and furious.

How can you tell if you've experienced a pregnancy nightmare? The dream will be dark, scary, filled with terrible images, and can very possibly cause you to cry or awaken suddenly. It's like watching a horror movie—about *your* life!

At such a happy time, why do we experience these terrible nightmares? They are a reflection of our anxiety, nervous anticipation, and worry about the pregnancy, the labor and delivery, and our ability to mother. They are *not* prophetic. During pregnancy, prophetic dreams always have a positive or happy energy to them, even if they are providing a warning about something. They will *not* inspire negative, pessimistic, or frightening images/ messages. Consequently, if a dream leaves you frightened, worried, pessimistic, depressed, or in some other negative frame of mind, it was a pregnancy nightmare.

Although you might be one of the rare women who do not experience pregnancy nightmares, they are so common that you might want to prepare yourself—and your husband. Unless your hubby has been deployed by the military or is a salesman who travels like mine did, he's probably going to be snoring peacefully by your side when you wake up from one of these scary dreams. Because you'll naturally gravitate toward him for comfort and reassurance, make your husband aware that these dreams have nothing to do with *him*, but instead are the result of hormones, worry, and nervous anticipation. Tell him that from time to time, you're going to need the comfort that only he can provide. When he cradles you in his arms you'll feel much better. Although it will take a little while to erase some of the very disturbing images that you'll see in your mind's eye during the nightmares, tell yourself that what you dreamt was absolutely nonsensical.

My Worst Nightmare

In my third trimester, when I was eight months pregnant with our son, I dreamt that I was back in Chicago where I grew up. I was dressed in a heavy winter coat and I stood on a deserted city street eerily illuminated by an overhead streetlight. It was late at night in the middle of winter, a frigid wind was blowing, and big snowflakes were swirling wildly around me. My son Flynn had already been born, and I was protectively cradling his tiny infant body. I suddenly looked down at him. In spite of the frigid temperatures, my infant son wore only thin, filthy, tattered rags. His body was pitifully grey and shriveled. My child had starved to death and it was my fault—because I forgot to feed him!

I awoke with a start. By then, accustomed to those nightmares, I chose not to wake my hubby, who was sleeping peacefully. Crying, I hoisted myself out of bed, waddled into the kitchen, and had a Haagen-Daaz moment. After I polished off an entire pint of chocolate-chocolate chip, I went back to bed and slept contentedly through the rest of the night.

ELEMENT TWO: CATEGORIES OF INFORMATION

Literal

When you receive literal information in a dream, the dream is easy to interpret. It is conveying *exactly* what you see, hear, or sense. For example, let's say that you are planning a surprise birthday party for your husband. The night before the big event, you dream about how surprised he was and how much everyone enjoyed the celebration. The dream was literal in nature because it conveyed information that was immediately understandable. In a literal dream, no interpretation is necessary. Although it's unconnected with pregnancy or conception, one of my very favorite stories, *A Christmas Carol* by Charles Dickens, provides a perfect example of a literal dream depicting what Scrooge experienced with the three spirits on Christmas Eve.

Symbolic

In a symbolic dream, you may "see" pictures in your mind's eye, or hear glimpses of confusing sounds. You may encounter symbolism, such as numbers or letters, snippets of music, or other sounds or images that initially make no logical sense.

For example, let's say that your doctor has told you that your due date is the very end of September. Your sister, who lives across the country, is planning to take time off of work to help you right after the birth, but she can only take ten days off and has to plan her vacation well in advance. You begin to fret about when she should take the time off to be of greatest help to you. Suddenly, you start dreaming about two symbols—the number ten and the number six. Every time you close your eyes, you keep "seeing" the numbers ten and six. It would very likely be the answer to your dilemma; the baby is going to come on October 6! Or say that you have a big fight with your husband and you feel miserable, wondering if you still love him. He tries to make up, but you reject his efforts. That night, in a dream, you revisit your lovely wedding day and hear snippets of a special song that was playing. You wake up realizing how much you still love your hubby and how much the relationship means to you. That kind of dream would occur to provide a terrific reality check.

Or let's say that you live in downtown Chicago and you spend all of your time in the city. Just before the holidays, you are working on a very important project at work that is highly stressful, labor-intensive, and time-consuming. You begin to wonder if you will finish the project before you give birth. That night, you have a dream about a white horse running across a daisy-strewn, hilly meadow. As a city dweller, that dream would not initially make sense to you—you do not own a horse, nor do you ever visit the country, nor is it summertime. But when you explore the images further, you'd realize that the dream was a respite, a getaway of sorts that was meant to be rejuvenating and recharging. The dream occurred for two reasons: first, it was meant to lift your spirits by allowing you to spend time in a warm, peaceful, and tranquil environment; and second, the dream was telling you—through its positive images and "feel"—that you were indeed going to successfully complete the project at work. This kind of symbolic dream is meant to be calming, restorative, and encouraging.

Or say that you love jazz and you have a dream in which you hear snippets of country music, sung by a female singer. Then the following day, you hear that the country singer you dreamt about had given birth the night before! The dream would have been conveying prophetic psychic information about someone whom you'd never even met!

Most human beings have symbolic dreams all the time. However, while you're pregnant, because your intuitive ability is so pronounced and you are more psychically sensitive, you're going to awaken many mornings full of questions as to what the dreams were trying to tell you. Symbolic dreams require interpretation. So what is the purpose of symbolic dreams if they're a bit challenging to decipher? Your angels often provide imagery or symbolism to promote your ability to conduct some spiritual work while your brain is shut down, as it is during sleep. You also receive symbolic information as a kind of reality check to help you remember to "bloom."

For instance, imagine that you are feeling horribly stressed because your mother keeps telling you what to do—or perhaps she criticizes your decisions. When mom tries to give advice, you bristle, and an argument ensues. Then let's say you have a symbolic dream in which you are at your mother's funeral, crying over the fact that you and mom had become estranged because of the bickering that resulted from her controlling behavior. At the funeral—in your dream—you are suddenly filled with an awareness about how you could have set more effective boundaries to create a better relationship with mom before she passed. You'd probably awaken from this symbolic dream a little frightened because you "saw" mom's funeral. At the same time, you'd possess an awareness of how to improve a relationship with an important spiritual student—your mother.

When I was pregnant with my son Flynn, I was trying to eat as healthfully as possible and avoid some of the foods I was really craving. One night, I experienced a dream in which I had given birth to twins—Oscar Meyer and Sara Lee!

When you have symbolic dream, evaluate the information

presented that you saw, heard, felt, smelled, or even tasted! Don't forget that we all receive very valuable information and messages at night when we sleep. I've discovered that when you write down the elements or dynamics of a dream, the pieces often start to come together. If you try to evaluate a dream, but do not feel that you've been successful with its interpretation, simply ask your unborn baby or angels what the dream was supposed to tell you.

ELEMENT THREE:
HOW YOU WILL RECEIVE
INFORMATION IN A DREAM

Lucidly

A lucid dream is best defined as being mentally alert or having cognizant awareness that you are, in fact, dreaming! In a lucid dream, you can receive information through literal or symbolic means. However, as you're receiving the information or messages, and the dream is running its course, you will have a conscious awareness that you're experiencing a dream. A good example would be a dream in which you receive a tangible visit from your unborn baby, guardian angels, or a departed loved one. In the dream, you realize that you are dreaming—at the very same time that you are aware you're conducting a very lucid conversation. When you wake up, happy and refreshed, you have a sense of *knowing* that you were really interacting with that spiritual being, rather than just a dream about them, and you'll look forward to the next visit! Not surprisingly, you are more likely to have total recall of a lucid dream than any other.

Seeing Images in Your Mind's Eye

Many of your dreams will be filled with breathtakingly vivid pictures and images that you can clearly "see" in your mind's eye. While you're pregnant, these dreams will be more vibrant and colorful than ever before. For example, in a dream you might visit a flower garden, the seashore, or find yourself on a mountaintop. Or you might clearly "see" another human or spiritual being in a dream. Or you might find yourself at the scene of an important event—past, present, or future—that you were meant to become aware of. If you do not see a crystal-clear image of someone or something in your dream, that means that the image was *supposed* to be fuzzy, clouded, or shadowed. Anything that is undistinguishable or out of focus is usually just a backdrop for more important elements of the message.

Hearing Sounds

During pregnancy, I believe that all of your senses become more acute, and your elevated hearing ability translates into your dreams as well. Once asleep, you might hear sounds—either accompanied by visual images or by themselves—that include conversation, music, laughter, weather patterns (such as a thunderstorm), animals (such as a dog's bark), chiming bells, the ticking of a clock, a vehicle's engine, footsteps, or sounds that remind you of a particular place, such as dreaming about Disney World where you went as a child. In dreams, sounds are as telling as visual images and provide just as much information.

Smelling a Scent or a Fragrance

In a dream, you might smell flowers, perfume, fresh paint, or the pungent docks on San Francisco's Fisherman's Wharf. Or, the smell of food—like home cooking—might alert you to the presence of a departed loved one. When I was pregnant, I often dreamt about my grandmother, Nani, and I could smell her Swedish pancakes, which I always adored as a child and now make for my own family.

A lovely man who attended one of my California workshops shared a very poignant story with me about the phenomenon of being able to sense a distinct smell in a dream. His twenty-two-year-old younger brother had been killed as a soldier in Iraq. The family wanted his services to reflect the young man's laid-back, youthful, and mischievous personality, but they were at a loss as to how they could create that atmosphere at a funeral. The night his brother's body was flown home, the man at my workshop told me that in his dreams, he clearly smelled the tantalizing aroma of In-N-Out, which is a casual, popular California eatery that serves hamburgers. When he awoke, he believed that his brother—through the dreams—was reminding him of how much he had adored those burgers, and he was providing a solution to the family's dilemma about the funeral. Because of that dream, the family had In-N-Out cater the services, which was a perfectly fitting celebration of that young man's life.

Physical Exertion

No matter what the state of your prenatal health, you will probably have dreams in which you are involved in arduous physical activity, like flying, jumping out of an airplane, running, gardening, swimming, riding horseback, bicycling, playing a sport, or even cleaning. Have you heard stories about people who do not have the use of their legs, but in their dreams, they are completely mobile and vigorous? So if you are forced to spend a part of your pregnancy in bed, these dreams might occur to help you feel invigorated—just like if you actually engaged in a form of physical exertion!

I've also found it very interesting that occasionally, after a very physical dream, I've awakened to discover that my feet and legs were actually *sore*—as if I had been tangibly involved in the forms of activity that I was dreaming about—while lying comfortably in bed! Has that ever happened to you?

Touching or Being Touched

Perhaps no other kind of dream experience will seem as tangible as when you're touching someone or they're touching you in a dream. While in a dream, you might "feel" the touch of your baby, a kiss from a departed loved one, or one of your angels might gently brush the hair from your eyes. Touching someone or something can be very emotional and allow a dream to be extraordinarily riveting and poignant.

The dreams about spiritual beings will take place because they wish to make their presence known to you as a form of support, or at those times when they're trying to convey an important message. The dreams about human beings will take place generally because a person has been on your mind, or because you're receiving psychic information about them regarding something that is very likely to take place in the future. While you're pregnant, you'll probably have many wonderful dreams that include your baby. When you wake up, you'll be convinced that the tangible interaction really took place!

Although it's not related to pregnancy, one of my favorite stories about having physical contact with a spiritual being in a dream was shared by a channeling client who was a fifty-five-year-old widow. Right before her birthday, she had asked her departed husband to make his presence known to her in some way because she missed him so much. The following night, she had a dream about him. In the dream, he took her out for a candlelight dinner, then they went dancing on the beach, and all of that was followed by intense lovemaking that was incredibly real and satisfying. She swears it was so tangible that she *knew* she was dreaming about the present, and that her sweetie had truly come to visit—and they were able to make love once again—in spite of the fact that he was in spirit!

Hearing a Voice Outside Your Head

In addition to receiving telepathic messages *inside* your head, you may also hear voices *outside* your head—as if another human being was speaking to you. This means that you'd be able to hear the actual voices of your angels, departed loved ones, and unborn baby—who, by the way, will use the voice that he will have as a child. When this occurs, it's really a fabulous sign that you are developing your channeling skills. It can happen when you're fully asleep, or when you're just coming out of a dream state. You'll be awakened by hearing your name called very softly, in soothing tones. Bleary-eyed, you'll probably look around and see no one there, but at the same time, you *know* what you heard. If the thought of communication this tangible appeals to you, simply *ask* the spiritual beings around you to communicate with you—with their own voices—outside your head. However, I have a suggestion. When I was pregnant with my daughter, Megan, I asked her to speak with me outside of my head in a way that was very clear and unmistakable. That night, after I had fallen asleep, I was startled awake by a thunderous voice right next to my ear exclaiming, "MOM! IT'S ME! MEGAN! I'M HERE!" She scared the dickens out of me! So if you ask for communication when you're sleeping in the form of a voice outside your head, make certain you also ask that the voice be a soft, gentle one!

ELEMENT FOUR:
HOW YOU WILL DREAM ABOUT TIME

References to timing, or time frames, will frequently play a part in your pregnancy dreams. Timing is extremely important! In your dream, you might "see" the pages of a calendar, hear snippets of a conversation about a particular date, witness some sort of holiday celebration, or see weather patterns that will denote a season or a time of year. Dreams frequently provide information or messages that reflect a specific time frame to alert you to something you have to accomplish by a certain date, prepare you for an event that's going to take place, predict when a loved one might recover from an illness, or answer a question you have about the timing of something—like the upcoming birth of your baby.

For example, after my family sustained damage in Hurricane Ike, we asked contractors to appraise the damage. They discovered that our air conditioning system was okay, but there were problems with the heating unit. I wasn't too concerned about it because we live in Houston, Texas, and it's generally very warm throughout the year. However, that night I had a dream about very inclement weather, and I could "see" my family shivering with cold. In the dream, I was receiving the message loud and clear that we needed to replace the heating system *right away*. Although this made absolutely no logical sense to me, and we were strapped for cash because the insurance company hadn't yet sent a check, we figured out a way to get it done. Three nights later, Houston was hit with unexpected record low temperatures—

twenty-eight degrees fahrenheit—and snow flurries! If we hadn't fixed our heating system, we wouldn't have been able to stay in the house and we might have had serious damage to our plumbing. I've learned over the years—inside and outside of pregnancy—to pay close attention to the time frames presented in dreams because they can be an integral part of the message that spirit is trying to communicate. For instance, if we hadn't quickly taken action to get our heating system repaired, we would have been ignoring the most important dynamic of the whole dream!

ELEMENT FIVE: WHY YOU REMEMBER SOME DREAMS WHILE YOU QUICKLY FORGET OTHERS

Some dreams are designed to be so unmistakable that you'll remember them without any problem at all, especially if the dream's purpose was to convey important or vital information to you. Even if the images are symbolic and you don't immediately grasp or understand the dream's meaning, you will remember it. Those are the dreams that register on your emotional radar screen because they're occurring for a specific reason: prompting you to take some action, protect your health or safety, answer a question you have, provide a reality check, or simply help you recharge.

Other times, you may not remember having any dreams at all, or you will not be able to recall what the dreams entailed. In this instance, it was unnecessary for you to remember the dream or have any conscious knowledge of it—because these were not forms of messages or information, but rather indications that your soul was conducting necessary filing. As we explored in previous chapters, your soul is an intricate computer that stores a journal of everything you have said or done in all of your lifetimes. Similar to saving computer files on a regular basis, your soul saves a diary of your experiences in this lifetime at night while you sleep. When this is taking place, you may see vague images in your mind's eye or hear things that are just out of earshot, and it may seem like a confusing hodgepodge of psychic images. This explains why you could have slept peacefully all night, and yet awakened tired. Your soul was hard at work! When your soul is conducting its processing, you will not have any recall whatsoever about what you've dreamt. And that's perfectly okay!

The way to make an easy distinction between dreams that occur to provide necessary information from those that reflect your soul's filing activity is very simple: the dreams you need to heed are those with clear images, sights, and sounds; involve timing; or have any other features that are focused and unmistakable. The dreams that are reflected by your soul's filing will be fuzzy, unclear, confusing, impossible to discern, and will not stir any kind of noticeable emotional reaction. You'll simply feel tired when you wake up.

ELEMENT SIX:
WHAT TO DO WITH PSYCHIC
INFORMATION OBTAINED IN DREAMS

There are two kinds of psychic information you will receive in dreams. First, you will obtain information that pertains to *you*. Second, you will be given information that pertains to *someone else*. All of this psychic information comes from your soul, unborn baby, angels, and departed loved ones. The spiritual beings around you are always in the process of sharing valuable intuitive messages that can help you get your life on track and moving forward with purpose and resolve. Prophetic, or clairvoyant, dreams typically focus on the present or the future. When one of these dreams occurs, it's important to pay close attention to the information contained in the message—as well as the time frames involved, if that was also a facet of the dream—and take whatever action the dream has indicated. Once you've awakened, if you're having trouble deciphering the meaning of a psychic dream, simply ask your unborn baby, guardian angels, or departed loved ones and they can fill you in. However, when you receive psychic information for or about others, the protocol can get a little complicated.

In my channeling workshops, people always ask about the psychic etiquette of a situation in which they've received intuitive information about another person. Should the information be divulged? This is something that each individual needs to decide for herself. However, my rule of thumb is this: if it involves someone's health or safety, I would share the psychic information, even if it makes no logical sense to you. For instance, let's say that you had a dream which indicated that your sister—a police officer—was going to be attacked at lunchtime in the parking lot of the police station. That would seem preposterous. Therefore, you might assume that you got the message wrong somehow. It's very common for people to dismiss the psychic information they've sensed, heard telepathically, or "seen" in a dream because on a surface level it strikes them as totally illogical. As a psychic, I frequently receive information for myself and others that initially appears illogical—but that's never prevented something from happening! And, understandably, when someone tries to interpret a psychic dream, they often worry, *but what if I'm wrong?* So, let's imagine that you chose to dismiss the psychic information about your sister's attack, and then it really happened? How would that make you feel? You might have been able to help her avoid the situation.

Another example: you dream that your mother-in-law has a small, contained malignant tumor in her breast. You'd probably feel scared, depressed, and very hesitant to share such negative information with her. Plus, you'd have to explain where you obtained this tidbit of psychic awareness. Therefore, because the situation was so awkward, you decide not to tell her about the dream. Then, six months later, your mother-in-law goes for her annual mammogram. The doctors find the tumor, but it has spread to her lymph nodes and is metastasizing. They tell her that if she had come in six months earlier, they might have been able to remove the cancer before it spread. How would you feel *then*? It's much easier emotionally to share intuitive information the moment you receive it, regardless of how you think the other person will react, rather than allow time to pass and a situation to possibly worsen. Interestingly, one of the primary reasons you'll receive intuitive information about someone else is because that individual has not been "hearing" the messages from their unborn baby, angels, or departed loved ones. Therefore, the spiritual beings ask you to be a messenger for them in the hopes that the individual might be more willing to "hear" another human being. This is why you may have experienced a situation in which you've spontaneously said something, and then immediately wondered, *where did that come from?*

Cheryle's Story

My daughter, Angelle, was extremely close to her paternal grandmother, Bevly. Bevly babysat Angelle from her birth until she was four years old so my husband and I could work. My daughter took it very hard when her beloved grandmother passed away in 2006. Bevly was survived by her husband, Louis.

When Angelle decided to get pregnant for the first time, she conceived without any problems and had a healthy baby girl she called Jordan Leigh.

During the time when she was trying to conceive again, she began to cramp and had a very heavy period. Her grandmother Bevly came to her in a dream and told her she had suffered a miscarriage. Bevly also reassured her that she would get pregnant again and have another child.

Angelle did get pregnant with her second child, but no one knew about the pregnancy except for her dad and me. She hadn't yet begun to show.

Meanwhile, her grandfather, Louis, became very ill and fell into a coma. He was rushed to the hospital and remained there for two weeks. When he finally awoke from the coma, the first thing he asked his son, Kenny—Angelle's father—was "How is the baby?"

Kenny naturally thought he was referring to the other grand-children, so he named them off one by one and reassured his dad they were all doing fine. Louis kept shaking his head and repeating in an adamant tone, "How is the baby doing?"

Finally, Kenny asked his dad, "You mean the baby that nobody knows about?" Louis nodded and answered, "Yes."

We believe that when Louis was in his coma, he saw and spoke with his departed wife, Bevly. They had always been very much in love and had been very close. We feel that Bevly told him about the baby.

Before Angelle had her second child, Louis passed away. Angelle's due date was May 18. Angelle would talk to her unborn son and ask if it were possible for him to be born on Bevly's birthday, which was May 1. Because Angelle loved her grandmother so, she thought it would be wonderful for her son and her grand-mother to have the same birthday. We all thought that it would be really nice, but highly unlikely since Angelle's due date was almost three weeks later.

May 1 started out like any other day. Angelle went to work as usual. Around midmorning, all of that changed. Jackson Marc was born that evening around 8:00 PM, on his great-grandmother's birthday. What makes our story even more remarkable is that Jackson is the spitting image of Angelle's grandfather Louis—who was the love of Bevly's life.

WHY YOU HAVE RECURRING DREAMS

Have you ever wondered why you've had *recurring* dreams— either inside or outside pregnancy? There are basically three different reasons for recurring dreams. First, you might be struggling with a fear or concern that has remained very stressful to you. That ongoing stress often results in mental fear-based dreams that are not intuitive and provide nothing more than a release—like a pressure cooker letting off steam. As long as you struggle with a particular fear, the dreams are likely to continue. Second, your soul wishes to get your attention about a particular issue you should be addressing, and it will continue to provide the same dream scenario until you understand what it is that you could be working on. Third, a recurring dream is coming from your unborn baby or guardian angels and is meant to create an awareness about something that is already happening behind the scenes or going to happen in the near future. We will often continue to have the same dream over and over until we can correctly interpret what the dream is meant to tell us.

The following true story was shared with me by a father who accessed prenatal intuitive messages from his unborn son:

Shannon's Story

Before my son Colby was born, I began to experience a recurring dream. It was always the same. It took place on a beach in Western Australia. In the dream, I was in a casual conversation with my lifelong friend Ted about a house he was building. Ted left to get busy on his house with two of his other friends.

Up from the water's edge came a tall young man who looked quite a bit like me, except for the fact that he had dark hair. (My hair is blonde/light brown.) I asked, "Are you one of Ted's friends?" And he replied, "No, I am your son."

I have always been able to "see" intuitively, but I never had anyone before in my life with whom I could share this connection until my son, Colby, was born. When he was a child, he would talk about his experiences with his "imaginary friends," and I totally understood. My return favor to my young son was to comfort him when others would tell him to "stop lying" or "making things up."

He is now grown, and throughout our entire lives we have been very close. Many people comment that we're like best friends. And, today, Colby looks exactly like he did in the recurring dreams I had about him before he was born. I believe my introduction to him years before my wife conceived allowed me to move forward to fulfill the destiny between us.

DREAM JOURNAL

I highly recommend that you maintain a dream journal to record all of the amazing information and messages you receive while you're expecting. Get a big notebook and divide it into three sections, one for each trimester of your pregnancy. When you have a dream, record the date and a description of what you "saw" and "heard." Then try to analyze the dream by using the template below:

Dream Journal

First Trimester

Date:

Description of my dream:

How did the dream make me feel? Who did I "see" or interact with in the dream? Was it a lucid dream? Did the dream involve messages from my unborn baby, guardian angels, departed loved ones, or my soul?

Was the dream literal or symbolic?

If symbols or images were present, what do I think they meant?

Was it a valuable spiritual dream or a fear-based nightmare?

What did I see, hear, touch, smell, or taste in the dream?

Did I hear a voice outside my head?

Did I perform any kind of physical exercise? Did the dream urge me toward completing some task?

Did the dream prompt me to begin a new challenge or project?

Did the dream urge me to share a psychic message with someone else?

Were there any time frames discernable in the dream? Is this a recurring dream? Why do I keep having it? If it was a fear-based dream, why do I think it occurred? What prompted the dream? What am I really worried about right now? What were the negative, worrisome, or frightening aspects of the dream that made it a non-prophetic nightmare?

After you've suffered a pregnancy nightmare, consider doing something dynamic and proactive to regain your emotional equilibrium. Get out of bed without waking your sweetie, grab a notebook, and write about the dream while it's still fresh in your mind. Then repeat the following mantras, or feel free to create your own!

My husband loves me. My husband and I will always share a happy, lifelong marriage.

I am going to be a wonderful mother.

My baby chose me because he has faith in me.

My baby will have food, clothing, and shelter.

I have lots of love to share with my baby.

My baby will know that he is loved and cherished.

My baby will be very happy that he chose me.

My husband will love our baby.

My husband will be a terrific father.

What my husband and I decide is the best decision for our baby.

The labor and delivery will be manageable.

The baby will continue to be in good health during the pregnancy. The baby will continue to enjoy good health after he is born.

The baby will be healthy even if I do not breast-feed.

I am in good health.

My husband is in good health.

This is the happiest, most exciting time in my life.

I am creating a miracle.

I have never been so beautiful.

You might consider printing these mantras so you have a copy by your bed and a copy you can carry in your purse for those less-than-confident, fretful pregnancy moments when you're suddenly wondering, "Oh-my-God-I-don't-know-if-I-can-do-this!" and "If-I-don't-breast-feed-will-my-baby-really-be-destined to-become-a-ruthless-desperado?" and "Are-we-going-to-be-financially-okay?" and "How-much-bigger-are-my-breasts-going-to-*get*?" and "How-*is*-this-great-big-baby-going-to-exit-from-such-a-tiny-narrow-orifice?" and "How-long-will-it-take-me-to-lose-all-the-baby-weight?" and "After-the-birth-will-my-vagina-be-so-big-that-it-will-accommodate-an-aircraft-carrier?" and "Will-I-really-be-able-to-learn-how-to-care-for-my-baby-after-he's-born?"

When I was pregnant with my daughter, I loved decorating her room—especially while I was nesting in my third trimester. After I'd awaken from a nightmare, my husband would find me sitting on the floor of Megan's nursery happily painting her furniture at 3:00 AM. Some postnightmare activities that you might want to consider if you can't sleep:

- Make an entry in your Dream Journal
- Write a special letter to your soon-to-be-born baby telling him or her about how you are feeling and all of the wonderful things you plan to do once the birth takes place
- Play with your baby's things, like his clothes, toys, books, mobile, etc.
- Eat something you love
- Pick up a positive book or magazine and read for a few minutes

- Take a shower and apply some body lotion
- Apply a facial mask and put oil on your cuticles
- Watch a film that makes you feel good
- Write a letter to a loved one
- Write thank-you notes to those who have been especially supportive
- Return e-mails
- Practice channeling with the baby, your angels, or departed loved ones
- Reorganize your drawers, cabinets, or closets
- Find great bargains on the internet
- Blog a pregnancy website
- Plan a last-time-we're-going-to-be-alone-getaway with your husband during your second or third trimester

EIGHT

YOUR UNBORN BABY CAN TELL YOU WHAT YOUR DOCTOR MAY NOT KNOW

Chapter Profile: Don't be surprised to "hear" messages from your unborn baby that might completely confirm—or surprisingly contradict—what your prenatal caregiver predicts about your due date, the weight of the baby at birth, or even its health! I wrote this chapter to provide food for thought about how "on target" the information really can be from your future offspring.

W hen it was finally time for my first prenatal appointment, I had no idea what to expect. My husband Britt took a seat while I approached the front desk at Dr. Schnider's office and signed in. I was at the opposite end of the emotional spectrum from only six months earlier when I had fled the same office in tears. The receptionist opened the glass window and welcomed me.

"We're pregnant!" I announced buoyantly.

"Congratulations," she smiled. "You picked a great OB/GYN. Dr. Schnider was just recognized by the *Best Doctors in America* publication. We're all very proud of him."

"That's wonderful," I said.

"So how is the pregnancy going?"

"I feel fantastic!" I told her. "And I can't *wait* to get my maternity clothes . . . but I guess I should hold off for another couple of weeks?"

She glanced at my flatish tummy and grinned.

"I wish I would begin to show," I said wistfully, gently rubbing my abdomen.

"Oh, you *will*," she chuckled.

"I'm a little worried because we still haven't bought anything for the baby."

"You've got plenty of time," she told me. "Besides . . . you don't know the sex of the baby yet."

"Yes, we do," I shared excitedly. "It's a boy!"

"How do you know that so early?" she asked, puzzled.

"He told me."

"Who told you?"

"The baby."

The receptionist stared back at me.

"His favorite colors are blue and red," I went on. "So that's how we're going to decorate the nursery."

She continued to stare.

"He's going to love airplanes, and—"

I was suddenly bumped from behind. I turned to see a very pregnant woman who had approached to sign in for her appointment.

"I'm sorry," she apologized. "I've gotten really klutzy."

"That's okay!" I said, looking down at her swollen tummy. "I'm pregnant, too!"

"I'm anxious for my baby to get here," she said, rolling her eyes.

"What are you going to name your daughter?" I asked, sensing that she already knew the gender of her baby.

"Rebecca," she answered, furrowing her brow. "But . . . how did *you* know I was going to have a girl?"

"Because she just told me."

"Who just told you?"

"Your daughter," I replied. "She's around you all the time."

"How do you *know* that?"

"I'm a channel."

"A what?"

"I'm a kind of . . . psychic."

"Oh!" she exclaimed excitedly. "Well, my husband thinks I'm a little nutty—"

"Don't they always?"

She giggled, "—but I just *know* things about my baby! All this time I've been wondering if I was just imagining it."

"Your daughter, Rebecca, is already communicating with you," I pointed out. "You two are bonding. Right now, she's telling me that her favorite colors are pink and yellow."

"Yes, I *know* that," the woman gasped, her eyes tearing up. "While I was still in my first trimester, I made my husband paint the nursery in pale pink and soft yellow . . . and then I found this flowered wallpaper border that matches perfectly! My husband is worried in case it's a boy."

We both laughed.

"The boy is coming next," I intuited.

"Oh, my God!" she cried, laughing through her tears. "We already have three!"

"Kim?" called Janet, the nurse, standing at the door that led to the exam rooms. Britt jumped up from where he was seated to follow me inside.

"Good luck!" I said to the woman. She wished me the same.

Janet led us to an exam room that held an ultrasound machine which would allow us a first glimpse of the baby. Britt took a seat while the nurse weighed me, took my blood pressure, then asked me to disrobe and "empty my bladder" so I could provide a urine sample. She left the exam room, and I quickly did what she asked. We didn't wait long before there was a faint knock at the door. The doctor came in and met Britt for the first time.

"You know, Kim, you're going to be one of my oldest prenatal patients," said Dr. Schnider. "I've only had one other patient who was older when she delivered."

"I'm going to be the healthiest patient you ever had," I proclaimed.

"Today, we're going to check on fetal development," the doctor told us. "This will be done by inserting this small probe into your body. It's called a transvaginal ultrasound."

Britt came to stand by my side and tenderly took my hand. He gazed down at me lovingly. I smiled up at him. Janet stood by the machine and suggested we watch the screen. Suddenly, a tiny image took shape. To my utter astonishment, I could clearly see a beating heart! I was overwhelmed with emotion. Seeing my baby for the first time was an experience I knew I'd never forget. "There he is!" I squealed.

"He...?" asked the doctor, smiling warmly. "You want a boy?"

"We really don't care," I shrugged happily. "But that's what he told me."

"Who told you?"

"The baby," I explained. "He also told me that he'll be born in the middle of February, he'll be full term, he'll weigh over eight pounds, and that I'm going to deliver him vaginally."

"Well . . . let's *see* about the due date," said Dr. Schnider, reaching for a little round calendar that resembled a wheel. "By my calculations, you're going to be parents right around February 14."

"That's what the baby told me!" I said to Britt.

"Congratulations," said the doctor. "Any questions?"

"Yes," I replied, quickly sitting up on the exam table. "How soon can we start my epidural? How about right now?"

The doctor smiled. "You've already decided against a natural childbirth?"

"Natural childbirth is giving birth with no make-up on," I responded.

"We can administer an epidural as long as you get to the hospital in time," said the doctor. "But seeing that this is your first child, I'm sure that won't be a problem. You'll be in labor for quite a while."

"I've been thinking about that," I said, frowning. "I don't want to be in labor for a long time. I'm going to try hypnosis to speed things up."

Dr. Schnider didn't comment, but it was my impression that he was less than enthusiastic about whether it would help.

"We have a list of questions," said Britt, who began by asking about the prenatal infant CPR class offered at the Woman's Hospital.

As I listened to Britt and Dr. Schnider, my mind was racing. I was going to give birth in February. It seemed a long way off, like that expression "so close and yet so far." The next seven months would allow me plenty of bonding time with the little soul who was going to join our family. Although I already *knew* that my son and I were communicating, the confirmation of his due date provided exciting evidence of our tangible, budding relationship.

The nurse presented us with a copy of the ultrasound scan. I looked at the blurry image of our offspring and my eyes welled with tears. I was really going to be a mom!

That was a watershed event in my life, and many other magical moments have followed, all related to having my babies and raising them. And there will be many magical moments ahead for *you* to savor and experience. Being pregnant and having a baby is like nothing else in the universe. I wrote this book in celebration of those magical moments. In addition to creating the awareness about communicating with unborn babies, I was eager to share my positive experiences with conception and labor and delivery when I was at the "advanced" maternal age of forty-four with my first child and forty-five when my second little one was born. If having a baby is also your destiny, I wanted you to have some encouraging, constructive information at your fingertips, written by a woman *just like you* who has already experienced the blessed event.

There are growing numbers of women who are choosing to delay pregnancy, in many countries around the world, and medical technologies are keeping pace by offering patients increasingly sophisticated treatment options in the area of obstetrics and gynecology. Ironically, over the last twenty years, as the number of fertility procedures have skyrocketed in the United States, I've had a surge of female clients question, "Is it still *possible* for me to have a baby? Since I've talked to my doctor, read some books on fertility, and researched on the Internet, I've gotten really worried about my age. I'm so old . . . I'm thirty-six! Everything that I've seen is so *negative!*"

I truly believe that it was my destiny to have children later in life. Only then could I reassure other women that it was certainly possible. I gave birth twice in my midforties, with no fertility help, and I trust that my experience provides a terrific reality check for any woman who is yearning to get pregnant but afraid she might not be able to turn her dream into a reality, especially if she is in her upper thirties or early forties—the age at which current fertility statistics start to nosedive.

In my private channeling sessions, the moment a client discloses concerns about fertility, I simply ask her angels for the specific details of how and when she is likely to conceive. I often discover that her unborn babies are already hovering, eager to answer all of her questions, even years before she might get pregnant. If a woman is wondering whether or not she'll ever be able to conceive, the communication with her unborn babies can be so heartening, like it was for me right after the first time I saw the gloomy, depressing statistics in my doctor's office. Remember that the souls of unborn children do not "queue up," as they refer to it, around women who are not destined to give birth or adopt a child.

Don't forget that your unborn baby knows all of the dynamics of his destiny because he is the one who planned it! All of the true-life stories that are included throughout this book illustrate how much valuable information is conveyed in the initial bonding process—*before* the actual birth takes place. This precious bonding is the reason why so many women just know, or sense, the very moment they conceive, the specific gender of their unborn baby, that they will have twins, the baby's choice of a name, or even its favorite color. A pregnant woman can sometimes predict the day she will give birth, which may be weeks before or after the tentative due date set by her doctor—because her unborn baby is telling her what she needs to know about the impending miracle.

Debbi, whose story follows, describes how she learned about the shift in her due date, not from her healthcare practitioner but from her unborn daughter—who communicated with her in *two* languages:

Debbi's Story

My daughter Gwen was conceived in early to mid-October 2007. In early December I was sitting on the couch in the living room when I received a very clear message in Swedish, *Det är trångt härinne!* That means "It's crowded in here!" This was especially funny because I had not even passed the first trimester mark, and if anything, it was only going to get more crowded in utero as the pregnancy progressed. It was also funny because my native language is English, but my husband is Swedish.

I predicted the delivery date to be June 27, the time of Swedish midsummer. Later, in mid-June, I discovered that midsummer was actually Friday, June 20. I was confused because I had felt so strongly that my daughter was to be born on midsummer.

Meanwhile, my son, Lukas, had been sick since early June with severe pink eye, double ear infections, an upper respiratory infection, and then unexplained stomach cramping that would cause him to cry for hours. I then received an unmistakable "knowing" from Gwen that she would delay her birth until her brother was well again.

On June 26, I had to pick Lukas up early from school because of tummy cramps. I gave him two quarts of tummy tea and plenty of crystallized ginger candy. Lukas finally felt well by noon on June 27. I proceeded to go into labor after 3:30 PM that same day. Gwen was born at 7:41 PM. Big brother Lukas was definitely well! My midwife and pediatrician told me that Gwen showed signs of being a postdate baby, which leads me to believe that she had been due on midsummer, June 20.

Gwen smiles sweetly right before falling asleep, and she has done so since birth. Yesterday, she was looking directly at me and smiling. I was overcome with the well-being of one visited by an angel.

How can a soul that hasn't even been conceived provide information that your experienced, skilled physician doesn't know? After all, your doctor probably has an impressive, lengthy curriculum vitae, which is what doctors call their resume of academic and professional accomplishments. An OB/GYN's professional life is not a simple or easy one. Dr. Schnider, my obstetrician, told me that in the past twenty-eight years he has planned all of his vacations around his patients' delivery dates; and, like physicians who practice in other specialties, he has found it necessary to depart important family celebrations at a moment's notice when his beeper alerts him to a patient in need. I think that physicians like Dr. Schnider are the true definition of dedication. Imagine that suddenly your job demanded that you be on call around the clock, and whenever your beeper went off you actually *had* to respond and abandon *whatever* you were doing and rush to your office? I absolutely adore my work as a channel and author, but being on call twenty-four hours of every day does not hold much appeal for me. Frankly, I don't know where doctors get all of that energy. Perhaps they should find a way to bottle it and offer it to the rest of us?

I have a number of physicians who are channeling clients of mine, in traditional specialties as well as alternative fields. The great majority of them have told me that they base a portion of their initial patient diagnoses on what they feel and sense, and then follow up by utilizing tests such as ultrasounds, amniocenteses, urinalysis, blood work, and numerous other diagnostic procedures to provide empirical validity to what they intuited. If your doctor relies on intuition or gut instinct, then he or she is likely receiving communication directly from your unborn baby—just like you are!

Michele's Story

In the doctor's office when I was about to have an amniocentesis, I swear the baby told me not to do it. So I didn't. I told my husband the baby was telling me that everything was fine. I said, "We don't need this test," so we decided against it. Not sure if that was just me or the baby, but I was so *certain* that *he* was telling me he was fine. I was only sixteen weeks along at the time.

If you have a healthcare provider who relies *solely* on what can be proven through experience or empirical evidence, and is quick to dismiss your "intuitive feelings" about conception, pregnancy, or the delivery, be prepared to sometimes find yourself, a little more in-the-know than your physician about what is occurring with your health and your unborn baby's health—because medical tests can only provide a finite amount of information. Carol is a perfect example:

Carol's Story

When I was thirty-three, I became pregnant with my last child. I was diagnosed with gestational diabetes. At five months, I started having preterm labor and had to start seeing a specialist for high-risk pregnancies.

When I went in to see the doctor, she did an ultrasound, but she opted not to perform an amniocentesis because of my preterm labor. The doctor told me that my baby was not in very good shape. She advised me to seriously consider aborting my pregnancy because the ultrasound showed that the baby's kidneys were not inside his body cavity. The doctor told me she was very concerned that my baby was not going to live very long because of all of the kidney and bladder problems that were visible on the ultrasound. She suggested that I go home and think about my options, and stay on complete bed rest.

At the time, I worked as a mail carrier. I was the mother of a six-year-old and an eighteen-month-old. I simply couldn't fathom how I was going to stay in bed all day! Because of the news I had received, I was a basket case. I had no more than a week to make the impossible decision. But in that period, I had more dreams and telepathic voices inside my head than at any other time in my life!

During that week, when I was resting, I "saw" my unborn child—happy and healthy. And I saw that he was a boy. The intuitive visions I had about him, along with the communication I had from my angels, assured me there was absolutely nothing wrong with my son and that all would be well. In that week of trauma, I found absolute peace with my decision to proceed with the pregnancy.

My son was born healthy, and he has always been my happiest child. He is now a young man of thirteen, six feet tall, and he plans to become an aeronautical engineer. He has been, and always will be, a shining light in my life—and I could never imagine my life without him.

Carol had to make an all-important decision, but she wasn't alone. Her unborn baby was there to share vital information about his health that could not be ascertained through the sophisticated technology available to her doctor. It is with remarkable courage that Carol chose to look beyond the tangibles of medical science and instead put her faith in what she was sensing from her future son.

There are still other instances in which the information you receive from your unborn baby—before you conceive and during your pregnancy—may not always mirror your doctor's advice or fall into the realm of your healthcare provider's experience or expertise.

Tiffany's Story

When I was pregnant with my daughter Candace, I had a very vivid dream that she was born with a dark mark on her cheek and that her head was red. After I awoke, I believed that the dream about the dark mark was meant to get my attention somehow. I thought about it many times afterward, and I wondered if I should bring it up to my doctor, but I didn't know how without sounding like a weirdo.

During her delivery, my pelvis proved too small for the baby to fit through, so ultimately, the doctor had to perform a C-section to avoid infection. Candace was a very healthy baby, but her little head was red and bruised in one area from all of the pushing during labor. I have come to believe that my unborn baby was trying to alert me to the possibility of a C-section! When I was expecting, I never once thought my unborn child was trying to communicate with me, so that is something I will definitely remember during any future pregnancies.

In another true story, Ali was present while her daughter was struggling with a difficult labor. Her soon-to-be-born granddaughter told Ali that, in spite of her mother receiving medication to speed up the labor, she would not be born until her daddy arrived on the scene. Sometimes a baby has timing that a doctor can't predict:

Ali's Story

It was June 10, 2006, and I was in the labor room at a local hospital with my daughter, Susan, who was expecting her third baby, Tiana. It was fifteen years after the birth of her second child, and it was looking like it was going to be a long, hard birth.

We had arrived at the hospital around 8:00 AM, and it was now early afternoon without any progress. Our friend, Jeanne, was with us as we waited. Jeanne and I were there to support Susan. The baby's father, who was a recovering drug user, had relapsed and my daughter was uncertain as to whether she wanted him in the delivery room with her. So Neil, the father, was downstairs, nervously pacing in the waiting room, while we were upstairs with Susan.

The process was slow. Susan had dilated only two centimeters over several hours without any progress. She was getting tired and the medication to help her dilate wasn't working. Jeanne and I felt helpless watching her struggle.

Out of the blue, Jeanne asked Susan if she had talked to her unborn baby to ask why she wasn't coming. Because she was laboring, Susan's response was not enthusiastic. After Jeanne made the suggestion, I decided that I would attempt to speak with my soon-to-be-born granddaughter.

So I sat in the chair next to the bed and began what I hoped would be a conversation with Tiana. I closed my eyes and concentrated, and I started to ask the baby if anything was wrong and why she was not proceeding with her birth. Immediately, I heard, "I want my daddy here." The response was so loud and so clear that I was really shocked. So I asked again, "Are you sure that is what you want, Tiana?" And I heard clearly, "Yes, I want him here and I want him *now*. My Mommy is sad and I want him here."

It was certainly not the response I expected, nor was I sure that

I liked the idea. We were all angry with Neil for relapsing, especially during the week the baby was due. But Tiana had spoken with me and I wanted to honor her request—and at the same time, do anything I could to help my daughter.

I approached Susan's bed. She was on her side getting an epidural, so there was literally no privacy with the doctor and all of the nurses in the room. So I bent down and whispered in my daughter's ear, "Did you talk to Tiana?" and she surprised me by saying, "Yes." Unwilling to speak first, lest I be wrong, I asked, "So did I. What did you hear?" Her energy was so consumed with the labor that my daughter was only able to whisper, "She said to call Neil." So I repeated what I had heard. The moment Susan was between contractions, she picked up the cell phone and called him. Within seconds, Neil ran into the room. He had been waiting right outside the door.

Minutes later, Susan started dilating. The labor and dilation progressed very quickly. Tiana was born vaginally within an hour after our conversations with her. She was a healthy, vigorous, and beautiful baby.

Ali's experience reminds me of what Shakespeare wrote in his play, *Hamlet*, more than four hundred years ago: "There are more things in heaven and earth, Horatio, than are dreamt of in your philosophy." I've channeled for clients who were told by their healthcare practitioner that they could never get pregnant, and a short time later they were happily celebrating the birth of a child. The most skilled and experienced caregivers can find themselves very surprised if they ignore their gut instincts. Each patient is unique. Every pregnancy is different.

In the following story, Kathy was so certain about what her unborn grandson told her about his date of birth that she made a wager with the obstetrician—and won! Here is her story:

Kathy's Story

When my daughter-in-law Stephanie was pregnant with her first child, the doctor kept changing the due date. At first, the doctor believed the baby would be born on July 22. Then, after sonograms and measurements, he moved the due date up to June 26. Stephanie was considering inducement, but I knew it was too early and convinced her that her baby needed as much womb time as possible.

About the middle of June, I asked the baby, "When?" He answered very clearly, "July 7." I was driving at the time and I almost had a wreck from all the joy I was experiencing in that moment. When I shared what my grandson had told me, some family members were very skeptical but believed me because I was so positive about what I had heard.

When Stephanie went into labor and checked into the hospital early on the morning of July 6, her OB/GYN told her that the baby would be born that afternoon. I told the doctor that the baby wouldn't be born until the next day. The OB/GYN was so confident I was wrong that he made a wager with me—which I accepted!

Late in the afternoon, the doctor was still certain that the baby would be born that day. He gave Stephanie drugs to speed up the process. Then he was suddenly called across the hall for a problem that became an emergency C-section. The drugs that were administered had the opposite effect and put my daughter-in-law to sleep.

Some hours later, when the doctor had finished with the other patient, he returned to Stephanie's room. Her labor pains had just started up again, and she was almost fully dilated. Although it was already after 10:00 PM, the doctor remained convinced that the birth was still going to take place that day. But the baby would not come down all the way. So, after midnight, the doctor decided to help things along by applying some light suction on the baby's little head.

My first grandchild, Ethan, was born at 1:14 AM on July 7, weighing nine pounds. I was there for the whole process, and I got to hold him while he was still wet and sticky. I was kissing him and crying with incredible joy. I told him that I loved him beyond measure and would protect him to the best of my abilities. The nurse finally had to ask for him because I just didn't want to give him up!

Kathy had already started the bonding process before her grandson was born, and was obviously very confident about what she had "heard." Similarly, Camille, in the story below, trusted in her intuition. Like Camille, have you ever had the experience, regarding any area of your health, in which your doctor had found something that concerned him, but you just knew that you were fine . . . and your intuitive information was proven correct?

Camille's Story

I was thirty-three years old, married five years, and had just realized that I wanted a child. Since the age of twelve, I had been taking a specific drug for treating epilepsy. Over the years, the doctors had always cautioned me that if I ever decided to start a family, I should come to them in advance so they could prescribe a safer medication for the pregnancy. Of course, I didn't think that I would conceive the first time I wasn't taking precautions—but I did.

My consternation and anxiety were as high as my joy when I discovered that I was pregnant. By the time I was able to see my treating neurologist, I knew that any damage to the baby had already occurred. The particular side effect on a developing baby from the drugs I was taking was a cleft palate. I was told that I had to wait for the results of the ultrasound that they give between twelve to sixteen weeks. I was nervous and apprehensive going into the ultrasound, and even more concerned as I waited three weeks to hear back after the test.

One afternoon during this agonizing waiting period I had laid down for a rest and was, as usual, worrying about my growing baby as I drifted off. After my nap, when I was waking, the first thing I "heard" was a very clear, firm, and slightly exasperated voice saying, "Mom, I'm just fine." I was not aware that it was even possible for unborn babies to communicate with us, and I did not share this incident with many people at the time. Nonetheless, I awoke with a terrific sense of calm and confidence that continued right through to delivery.

We were blessed with a beautiful, healthy, extremely bright boy who is now eighteen years old. I *know* that it was him communicating with me all those years ago—because I've heard the exact same "exasperated" tone of voice . . . all throughout his teenage years!

It's important to remember that our physicians—no matter how much we respect, trust, and revere them—are mere mortals like the rest of us. We put such weighty responsibilities on their shoulders the moment we place ourselves in their care! There may be instances in which your intuitiveness alerts you to something long before medical testing can confirm it or a doctor can diagnose it. I've had the experience of channeling for people whose unborn babies or guardian angels have recommended that they go for medical tests because of a specific condition or as a preventive measure. On occasion, a client has called back and told me that the doctors could find nothing wrong. Why was that? Because angels and unborn babies can sometimes "see" things long before they can be picked up with even the most sophisticated medical equipment.

For example, have you ever experienced a strong, unmistakable feeling that something was going on inside your body, but your physician was unable to find anything wrong—even after giving you a thorough exam or prescribing various tests and procedures?

Maria's Story

Twenty-two days before my due date I was getting ready for a prenatal appointment. I was feeling great. Every day the baby vigorously kicked and was very active and my doctor gave me glowing reports each week. I had absolutely no reason to be concerned. As I was admiring my pregnant profile in the mirror, out of nowhere I heard the phrase, "something is not attached." I had no idea what that meant or why that popped into my head.

Later that day, the results of my prenatal appointment were fine. Although the baby had a strong heartbeat, I told the nurse that I was worried because of the telepathic message I received earlier. She said, "Why? Everything looks great."

That afternoon, I noticed a lack of fetal movement for the first time. The baby moved only once in a few-hour period. This concern was multiplied when I remembered the message "something is not attached."

I called my doctor and he said to track the baby's kicking through the night and let him know the next morning if there was no change in the amount of movement. The baby typically kicked all night long, but that night she moved only two or three times. I paged the doctor first thing the next morning. He asked me to come in immediately, and I was placed on the fetal monitor in the hospital.

They discovered that my baby was in major distress with an

extremely weak pulse, so an emergency C-section was performed. During the operation, I heard my doctor say, "The placenta is not attached. It has separated by 50 percent." Later, he told me that I was very lucky because my baby girl was scarcely breathing when she was born. Thankfully, she was breathing on her own after about ten days.

Now my baby is very alert and laughing and smiling all the time. And yesterday, she said "Dada" for the first time! I was very grateful to have received a heads-up from her before she was born, because I had heard so many times that the closer you get to your due date, the less movement there is due to the fact that the baby is getting so big. I would not have taken the decrease in movement as seriously had that ominous message not been relayed by her that day . . . with perfect timing. I believe that my unborn baby provided the message I needed to help save her life.

While it's true that physicians possess dedication, have the most advanced equipment at their disposal, offer patient treatment in clean, safe facilities, and possess the willingness to keep informed about ever-expanding medical technologies, there are still times when a physician can provide a completely different opinion about when a patient will go into labor and delivery than the due date determined by the unborn baby. This phenomenon happens all the time, so don't let it confuse you into believing that you didn't "hear" your baby correctly.

Tina's Story

My daughter Brandie was pregnant with her second child, and soon into the pregnancy I *knew* this baby was a girl. Like any grandparent or parent, we were prepared for either boy or girl, and our lives would have been blessed with either outcome. Deep inside, I felt like I knew this little soul already. Her energy was so powerful. Her mommy knew as well that this little one—baby Abbie—was going to come into this world much differently than her first child, who was a boy.

Complications began early in Brandie's pregnancy. All of the ultrasounds were showing what seemed to be a serious issue with the uterus. Starting in my daughter's twenty-eighth week, severe contractions were causing concern. Our natural fear of the baby being born prematurely started to overwhelm us. My daughter maintained the pregnancy to thirty-two weeks, and we were beginning to feel hope that Abbie was going to make it full term.

However, Brandie suddenly started to have contractions every three to four minutes over a five-hour period. The doctor immediately admitted her into the hospital and started medications to halt the contractions. My daughter and I both *knew* this child wanted to come meet her family earlier than the planned date—we could *feel* it. Over the next week, the contractions continued to be a cause of concern. The doctor prepared for a very serious delivery, with many specialists gathered to help him.

I have turned to Kim many times when I felt something on a gut level and needed intuitive validation. So, during our channeling session, I asked Kim if she could "see" if my grand-daughter, Abbie, was going to be born sooner than expected. With a very quick response, Kim assured me this little one was not going to wait until her September due date. Kim also spoke with the baby and asked her if she could wait until her little body could grow more before birth. Even before Kim could finish the question, baby Abbie was vehemently responding, "No!" This was the *exact* feeling I was getting from my granddaughter as well. Kim also referred to her as a little "fiery" soul. This, too, is the same energy I was feeling when I spoke to the baby. I could feel that Abbie wanted to be with us as soon as possible.

Kim told us to be sure that Brandie was in, or near, the hospital around August 10. Kim kept telling us that the baby would most likely be born on August 14, which was the date that my mother and best friend predicted early in the pregnancy. That would mean that Abbie would be arriving four weeks before her due date. I also asked if my daughter would have to have a hysterectomy, as the doctor had forewarned. Kim could see that other souls were already lining up to be part of Brandie's future family. At this point in the pregnancy, there seemed to be no possible way of saving the uterus. So when Kim "saw" another pregnancy, we were shocked to say the least.

Abbie was born on August 14. During the caesarian, when the doctor entered the uterus, he realized that it had a film, of sorts, over it—and that was what had looked like placental problems on the ultrasound. Brandie's uterus was clean and healthy. In fact, the doctor told us that in light of what he had seen earlier on the ultrasound, that he had never experienced this positive of an out-come in twenty-seven years of practice.

Our gorgeous girl created a situation that delivered her to us early, and yet caused no harm to herself or her mommy. We knew all along that our baby was coming early—we could *feel* it.

As I held my beautiful granddaughter for the first time, I felt that I already knew her. Just hours old, she gave me a smile when I said, "Hello, sweetheart—I am your Nani!"

As you take the journey down the magical path of having chil-dren, you might want to consider discussing what you have heard or sensed from your unborn baby or your angels with your OB/GYN—or any other healthcare provider for that matter—regardless of whether you believe they embrace spiritual sensi-bilities. Your health and that of your unborn child are at stake. Think of a doctor as your partner in helping you maintain your good health. When you receive intuitive information that you feel is vital for your physician to know, it's important for you to share and *feel* heard. It's up to you to assist those who are striv-ing to provide the best possible health care for you and your little ones!

How do you convey the intuitive information you've received to your doctor? This is really not a tricky situation at all—even if you suspect that your physician is not receptive to hearing about things that are spiritual in nature. Simply come right out and say, "Dr. Jones, my unborn baby has told me that . . ." Or, you could present the information in a more subtle way by saying, "Dr. Jones, I have been sensing that . . ." The most important thing is for you to feel *heard* by your provider.

Remember that your physician works for you and is there to provide the best health care possible. If there is a message you received from your unborn baby or guardian angels related to your health or that of your baby, then it is your responsibility to share it—as quickly as possible—with your healthcare provider. If it could prevent an unwanted situation from arising or help minimize a health situation that is not yet obvious, isn't it in your best interests to explore the messages from spirit so you can truly be a partner in your own health care?

Every so often in one of the in-person workshops I conduct around the United States, someone will remark, "I'll feel silly going to my doctor (or husband, mother-in-law, sister, etc.) and sharing a 'message' that I've received from a spirit!" To which I always reply, "And how would you feel if you received information from spirit, and didn't share it . . . and something were to occur that could have been prevented? Which would make you feel worse—feeling silly initially, or terribly regretful after the fact, knowing that you might have been able to prevent something unfortunate from happening?"

Remember that your baby can relay information unavailable to your physician because it is clairvoyant, which means that it is related to future events that haven't occurred yet and are beyond normal sensory perception. While it is true that your doctor has a wealth of experience and education to draw on, he or she maintains a focus on the here-and-now. With all due respect to your wonderful healthcare provider, I would argue that your baby may at times have a view of the bigger picture. Take that into account before you dismiss the channeled messages you are receiving.

For instance, when I was pregnant with my daughter, Megan, she told me she was going to be larger than her brother, Flynn, was at birth. When I shared that tidbit of information with Dr. Schnider during one of my prenatal appointments, he shook his head and told me that because she was a girl, she probably wouldn't be as big as my son, who had been born the previous year. Dr. Schnider went on to explain that I was so huge because I was expecting my second child and my tummy muscles had already been stretched. That made sense, too.

During delivery, however, when Megan was born, the intuitive information I had received proved correct. My infant daughter was twenty-two inches long and weighed nine pounds, three ounces—one inch longer and one full pound heavier than my son had been at birth.

NINE

UNDERSTANDING FERTILITY AND PREGNANCY CHALLENGES

Chapter Profile: I'm sharing a unique perspective on how timing impacts conception and birth. I explain the fact that a completely healthy pregnancy —like mine—could be considered "high risk," as well as true-life stories about women who became pregnant despite the odds against them. The chapter also features advice from a respected OB/GYN, an internist, a midwife, a hypnotherapist, and the angels with whom I've channeled about conception, and it explores what you can do to help ensure that your one-of-a-kind prenatal experience is as healthy and stress-free as possible!

Many years ago, I remember having dinner with a girlfriend who was complaining about how much work it was for her and her husband to conceive. I tried to be sensitive, but I couldn't relate to what she was talking about—at all! At the time, I was doing everything I could to *avoid* pregnancy.

How hard could it be, I wondered, once a person has finally met a Mr. Wonderful who miraculously rose to the occasion and proposed? No more sifting through all of the Mr. Wrongs, no more bad dates, no more romantic disappointments. Finding the elusive Mr. Wonderful was the hard part . . . and everything after that would be smooth sailing. You meet *The One*, you get married, you have great sex whenever you want, and then you decide if and when you want to start a family, and bingo! You get pregnant. The baby-making equipment is there, ready and waiting, entitling a woman to her own children when and if she decides that she's ready. What could possibly be so hard about *that*?

To be frank, at that time other people's children often annoyed me in grocery stores, the post office, in restaurants, and other public places when they'd scream, cry, shout, run around, sneeze plague-like germs in my direction, or worst of all . . . whine! In my twenties, I once babysat for a girlfriend who had two small toddlers. When my friend returned a few hours later, I was in a state of utter exhaustion . . . and ready to get my tubes tied. Afterward, I called my mom to complain about how much work it had been and how demanding the children were. She chuckled before quickly assuring me, "Don't worry honey, it's completely different when they're your own."

While some women are very mature in their twenties, I remained an adolescent bubblehead. I was struggling with a series of major personal issues, and it was all I could do to take care of *myself*. I wanted a baby as much as I wanted to take the next space shuttle to the moon. So during the years when many of the women I knew were starting families, I reasoned that it would be wise to put off having a child until I met Mr. Wonderful, established my profession, and reached a higher level of emotional and spiritual stability. I figured that I'd *know* when the time was right for me. Throughout my twenties and thirties, I remained skeptical as to whether I would ever be able to create that perfect scenario, and it continued to seem unattainable and out of my reach.

Fast-forward twenty years. I had just married Mr. Wonderful. My career was established, and through therapy and hard work I had resolved my serious issues. Suddenly—seemingly out of nowhere—a desire bubbled up inside of me. I yearned to have a baby! I never realized how primal an emotional feeling could be. It was finally my time. I was in my early forties, felt young and hearty, had no health problems, exercised regularly, and took vitamin supplements. With emotions ping-ponging from gut-wrenching nervous anticipation to wild, confident exhilaration, I stopped taking the Pill for the first time since I was twenty-three.

As I shared in the first chapter, when I announced my joyful intentions to Dr. Schnider, an experienced OB/GYN and fertility specialist, he gently shared grim statistics about my chances of getting pregnant. I was shocked to learn that he considered me "high risk" just because of my age, in spite of the fact that I felt so strong and energetic.

It had truly never occurred to me that my fertility could have been slowly, silently ebbing away—not as long as I was still getting my period. When my angel John and my unborn baby reminded me that destiny was to play a major role in my ability to become a mother, it allayed my fears, and I was positive and optimistic again. My husband and I got pregnant a few months later—with no fertility help from Dr. Schnider. I was overjoyed.

Four weeks later, in mid-December, my husband and I were listening to holiday music as we were joyfully decorating our Christmas tree, thrilled about all of the incredible blessings that were going to take place in the New Year. I suddenly started cramping and bleeding, and I ultimately had a miscarriage. My hormones had been charging upward in those precious few weeks of pregnancy, and now they were abruptly diving, plunging me into a black hole of hopelessness and negativity. To my astonishment, after I lost the baby, I discovered that life alone with my Mr. Wonderful just wasn't going to be enough. Every time I saw a pregnant woman or a mother with children, I would burst into tears and sob my heart out.

All during that period of anguish, I could sense my unborn baby hovering around me, but I was far too despondent and depressed to speak with him. I wondered why he maintained a presence following the miscarriage.

After I lost the baby, I continued to work full time channeling for others, and it was a godsend. It forced me to focus on other people and their challenges. After a few months, I was able to recapture a little emotional strength. So out of desperation—and curiosity—I began to speak with my unborn baby again.

At my invitation to "talk," he immediately apologized for what had happened. He told me that early in the pregnancy, he had suddenly become frightened about his ability to accomplish everything he had planned for his upcoming earthly lifetime, so he had decided to wait. He explained that his decision resulted in the miscarriage. I was shocked at what he told me, and naturally very hurt and angry that he would do that to me and my husband! I asked how it was possible for *him* to decide to end the pregnancy while he knew that I wanted it so badly, and at the same time my physical body remained in such perfect health.

My unborn baby explained that at any time during a pregnancy, a soul can change its mind and a miscarriage would ensue—without any discussion with his chosen birth mother. He explained that it is the personal prerogative of each soon-to-be-born soul to change its mind at any time during a pregnancy, if it felt concerned about its ability to achieve everything that it had planned for its upcoming earthly lifetime. The unborn baby's decision is unrelated to anything the birth mother does—or doesn't do—while she is pregnant. In this case, the birth mother is not responsible for a miscarriage.

Almost without exception, he said, that same soul will be born to the mother it had originally chosen, at a *later date*, to allow the soul extra time to review the choices he had made in regard to his spiritual agenda, or blueprint. This extra time is necessary when a soul becomes concerned about being able to achieve everything he had planned for his upcoming earthly lifetime. Rather than reinventing the wheel by altering his choices, the soul will maintain the same list of goals—but remain in heaven while putting finishing touches on his courage and confidence before taking the plunge. It is very much like climbing the ladder to the high dive, but then getting frightened once on the diving board. Because the whole key to success in developing enlightenment is centered on fulfilling one's spiritual blueprint, a soul may wisely decide to delay his earthly journey until he will have more success in accomplishing his spiritual objectives. My unborn baby then surprised me by pointing out that the mother has a similar prerogative because she can choose to terminate her pregnancy without consulting the fetus.

This revelation hit me like a bombshell. My stunned reaction was unrelated to my moral, ethical, or political sensibilities; all I could do was think about my dreams of having children and the way in which they had been shattered so abruptly. But then it slowly started to make sense. No wonder so many seemingly healthy pregnancies ended without logical medical explanation. And then I thought of how many of my clients and girlfriends who were expecting a baby had commented, "I have this *knowing* that the child I am pregnant with now . . . is the same child I miscarried last year!"

My unborn son promised that he would still come to me, but that he needed more time to get his plans in order related to his destiny. He told me that he had chosen February as the month of his birth, in the year of the dragon, per the Chinese calendar. I wanted to learn everything I could about this, so I made a quick trip to the bookstore. The time of the dragon was two years away, which meant that I would supposedly get pregnant again sometime during the next spring.

I began to talk to my unborn son every day, and he kept

reassuring me that once I was pregnant, he wouldn't change his mind again. I was very frightened but I chose to trust him.

True to his word, I got pregnant again in late spring of 1999, with no fertility help. I remained well and strong during the duration of the pregnancy. Our healthy little dragon, Flynn, was born February 18, via a vaginal birth that lasted a little over five hours. The moment he was born, I heard a little girl's voice inside my head: "I'm next, Mommy!" Fourteen months later, without any fertility help, I gave birth to a healthy nine pound baby girl we named Megan. I was forty-five years old. So take heart! It happened for me, and it can be possible for you, too! While I loathe statistics, I want to focus on them for a moment because you're going to be exposed to them everywhere. Approximately twenty-five percent of pregnancies end in miscarriage. I've had two miscarriages; one when I was in my early twenties at a time I was trying to avoid pregnancy but foolishly had not gone on the Pill yet, and then again when I was initially pregnant with Flynn. I'll bet that a lot of the women you know have had at least one such experience.

Michelle's Story

I'm reaching the end of my thirty-eighth week and today, for the first time, I had a connection with my unborn baby. I was resting when I heard a voice calling, "Mom! Mom!" I will never forget this. Since I have had a prior miscarriage, I had tears of joy. I can't wait to meet my child.

Although I was scared silly to repeat that horrible event and miscarry again, I choose—wholeheartedly—to take the risk. If I had listened to everybody who told me I was too old, or that the chances were high that I would lose another pregnancy, I wouldn't have given birth to my two babies.

By the way, were you aware that women who opt to conceive later in life have become the fastest-growing segment of the booming pregnancy market? According to a recent survey by the National Center for Health Statistics, future trends show that women will continue to delay motherhood. This phenomenon is sweeping other countries as well, including the United Kingdom, Australia, Sweden, and Japan.

Let's take another look at the statistics by reframing them. Although 25 percent of pregnancies end in a miscarriage, consider the fact that *75 percent* of pregnancies do *not* end in miscarriage. The *World Fact Book* estimates that more than 128 million babies will be born around the world . . . and that is in 2008 alone. That breaks down to over 353,000 babies born every *day* of the year!

Vinaya's personal experience chronicles how her future son helped her heal following a miscarriage.

Vinaya's Story

My first pregnancy ended in a miscarriage, and I was extremely depressed for quite some time. Then I got pregnant again. I was happy, of course, but also very nervous because of my previous experience.

One day when I was in a semiawake state, I "saw" a small boy of about three years old appear and tell me that he would soon be coming into my life. The image was crystal clear. I felt very blessed! From that time forward, I knew that my baby would be born without a problem, and that he was going to be a boy. My unborn son provided me with the calm assurance I needed to be able to relax, feel secure, and really enjoy every moment of the rest of my pregnancy.

The vision proved even more prophetic when, four years later, I realized that my son, who I had named Vikas, looked exactly the way he did when he first appeared in spirit form to support and comfort me.

In addition, women have been known to get pregnant with conditions such as endometriosis or intermittent ovulation, while on the Pill, after surgeries such as vasectomies and tubal ligations, without penile penetration, while using condoms, after the onset of menopause, by having intercourse with a partner who has a low sperm count, and following abortions, as well as following previous drug or alcohol abuse. Chances are you'll probably get pregnant, stay pregnant, and give birth without any truly significant complications. In fact, surprise pregnancies, like Nicola describes below, occur all the time.

Nicola's Story

Months before I became pregnant with my son Milan, I sensed his presence. I strongly felt a little soul wanting to be in human form. It was like he was talking to me, asking to be born to experience life on the earthly plane.

Milan's conception was a miracle in itself. There were no plans to have any more children, ever. According to my biological cycle, it was impossible for me to get pregnant at that time. So imagine my surprise when I found out that I was expecting. I was awestruck that this baby wanted to be born through me. It felt like an agreement—a bonding—between souls, and I embraced it.

From that moment on and throughout the pregnancy, I had a strong sense of knowing and connection with the soul that was going to be my new little baby. He slept when I slept, and he gently moved when I was awake. Whenever I touched my growing tummy, I felt this incredible energy and light between the baby and me. I had a wonderful feeling of knowing and a sense of belonging . . . which was an incredible sensation.

Our special connection has continued ever since. Milan, now in kindergarten, is wise beyond his years. He literally is an angelic old soul and enlightened in how he expresses himself, what he does, how he thinks, and how he interacts with others. These bonding experiences we had on my spiritual journey make me believe that all children/souls have an agreement with their birth mother.

DESTINY AND FERTILITY

Are you aware of the significant role destiny plays in your chances of getting pregnant and giving birth? Although you have to do your part to make things happen, the timing of a pregnancy is usually not determined by the mother or her physician—but the unborn child.

A woman can come to believe that she has fertility problems because conception isn't happening within *her* time frames, when in fact there are no fertility issues . . . it's simply that her baby isn't ready to come yet! Interestingly, if a child's destiny is to join your family through an adoption and he has planned to come first, then it is highly unlikely that you will get pregnant until *after* the adopted child has arrived.

Each soul that is planning to return to the earthly plane must choose his birth mother and father, his birth date and time, and his birth order in regard to his siblings. The soul makes those choices in an effort to create the most favorable opportunities to work through issues, achieve his life's work, and successfully interact with other souls who are also returning to the earthly plane. Therefore, for some women, pregnancy ensues when they are very young; for others, like me, it happens later in life.

My belief is that if having a child is your destiny, it *is* possible to make it happen. I fully understand how hard it can be to persevere when you've tried to get pregnant and it hasn't happened yet, or if you've experienced a loss such as a miscarriage or an unsuccessful in vitro. Each time you try to get pregnant, you're taking a risk. You could end up getting your period next month. You could get pregnant and lose the baby. Or, after surrendering your physical body and spending thousands on in vitro, you might fail to conceive for a while.

There is no question about the fact that it requires raw courage and resolve to make a baby. And it might be argued that the process of adoption takes even more perseverance. All of your heartfelt emotions, physical energy, and hopes for the future are at stake. Perhaps there is nothing that you'll try harder to achieve than to give birth to or adopt your children . . . if that is your destiny.

How do you *know* if something is predestined? Destiny refers to the general spiritual blueprint of your life. Destiny involves all of the opportunities that will prevail as you travel your life's path. How do you know which opportunities you can turn into a reality? Look inside your heart. What are the things that you most desire? What thoughts, ideas, or dreams make your heart and soul sing? More often than not, those things make up your destiny. Simply stated, it means that if you yearn for a baby, then it is likely that becoming a parent is part of your destiny.

We are all as individual as snowflakes in regard to our destiny, and that uniqueness is reflected in our choices. One of my single female clients chose to buy sperm from a reputable sperm bank in California and has happily given birth to two healthy sons. I also know a number of families who have chosen adoption. Others I know have chosen to buy eggs or use a surrogate. Still others have chosen in vitro fertilization.

At the same time, there are a growing number of people consciously choosing not to have children. My darling stepdaughter always *knew* that her destiny did not involve giving birth or raising children of her own.

Jennifer's Story

I am thirty-five and in perfect health. I have been married to the love of my life for eight years. I have a good career, a loving family and friends, and I have a home I adore. God could not bestow upon me any more gifts than I already have. I was never that girl who knew as a child she wanted children; I have never felt I would be incomplete without them. I have never longed for them or agonized over whether to have them. It has simply always been a truth inside my heart that I was not destined to live my life with children in my home, as gorgeous and blessed as I know all children are. I love children, and I am comfortable around them, as they are with me, but I am not a mother, and I love my life as it is.

Every human being has a different life plan that is perfect for them. And each individual knows what is best for him or her. You know what's best for you. Destiny will often dictate:

Your likes and dislikes
The direction in which your dreams and goals will take you
Life paths you will rightly reject as inappropriate for you—
    and the courage it will require to stand by your convictions

How events will unfold throughout your life

The timing in which those events will occur

WHY STRUGGLE IS NECESSARY

As you make your special and unique journey, you are certain—like everyone else on the earthly plane—to encounter *some* struggle. We all encounter some kind of challenge as we pursue various goals and dreams. Struggle presents an individual the opportunity to evolve spiritually and emotionally through experiencing adversity.

You may experience struggle as you attempt to have a family, while other women seem to get pregnant with no effort at all. Just because there is some level of struggle involved with having a family does not mean that it is not right for you, or that you can't possibly turn it into a reality. What's more, in addition to having children, there will be many other dreams you'll have in your life that represent *all* of the marvelous things you are destined to achieve.

It was Harriett Tubman's destiny to be born into slavery in 1820, in Maryland. It was her destiny, at thirteen, to sustain a head injury so violent that it resulted in epileptic seizures that would plague her for the rest of her life. Yet she was able to make a death-defying escape from slavery when she was twenty-nine. It was also her destiny to become a leader in civil rights by helping other slaves escape, and to work tirelessly for women's suffrage. It was Helen Keller's destiny to be stricken with a fever at eighteen months that left her blind and deaf before she had learned to speak. Yet it was also her destiny to graduate Radcliffe College cum laude and become a world-renowned author, speaker, and activist for the blind and hearing impaired. It was Florence Nightingale's destiny to be born into a wealthy, conservative British family in 1820, when women from upper-class backgrounds were expected to become wives and mothers. Over the strident objections of her family, she followed what she considered to be a divine calling in nursing, which at the time was considered by many to be a disreputable occupation. Instead of living in sumptuous wealth and enjoying her leisure, it was her destiny to devote her life to caring for the poor and advocating better conditions for those subjected to workhouse infirmaries. In 1854, accompanied by a small group of nurses, she traveled to Turkey to heal British soldiers who had been wounded on the front lines of the Crimean War. Her tireless efforts at the camp dramatically improved the survival rate, and she pioneered many of the modalities and techniques of modern-day nursing.

In the next true-life story, Lisa relays how she had the support of her best friend, Mary, during labor and delivery . . . in spite of the fact that Mary had died shortly before the birth:

Lisa's Story

I had a series of spiritual experiences with an old friend involving the birth of my son. I first met Mary when we were roommates at Southwest Texas University, and we became as close as sisters. Still the best of friends after graduation, we stayed in close contact. Back then, my intuition always told me when she was feeling depressed or worried, and I would pick up the phone and call her. After I'd question, "What's *wrong?*" she would laugh and ask me how I always knew when she needed to talk.

When I became pregnant, she was absolutely delighted for me. I was going to be a single mom, and as my best friend she told me that she *had* to be present when I gave birth. I assured her that she would be and that I really needed her with me. As the pregnancy progressed, Mary became more and more excited.

On the day of my big baby shower, Mary didn't show up. I felt incredibly hurt and puzzled as to why she would fail to attend such an important event in my life. My dear friend didn't even call to explain why she had chosen not to come. I couldn't get over it. She never contacted me, so I assumed that for some reason she decided to back away from our friendship.

The days flew by, and soon I was seven months pregnant. My tummy had ballooned, and I was still working full time. One day I came home from work really exhausted. My ankles were swollen and my whole body ached. I kicked off my shoes and started to relax in my favorite chair. The phone rang, and I was so tired that I didn't want to get up to answer it. My mother was visiting, so she reached for the receiver. I heard her gasp and suddenly say, "Oh no! Oh my God! When?"

I sat straight up and knew in that instant that something was wrong with Mary. Even though her name was never mentioned, I just knew. I got up and approached my Mom, asking, "What's wrong with Mary?" Mom's face wore a heartsick expression. She gestured for me to be patient while she kept talking on the phone. I felt a sickening dread in the pit of my stomach. My heart was pounding and I couldn't wait any longer, so I grabbed the receiver and asked, "What's wrong with Mary?"

It was Mary's mother. She told me that Mary had been shot. I immediately asked what hospital she was in. Her mother told me that she was dead. She had died the day of the baby shower! Mary's mother said that because I was pregnant, she had decided not to tell me until after I had given birth so as not to cause a miscarriage. However, she was now calling because she had to; the authorities were investigating Mary's death, and because we were long-standing friends, they might arrive on my doorstep to ask questions. Mary's mother wanted to relay the horrible news herself rather than my hearing it from the authorities. I literally fell to my knees sobbing.

When my water broke, I was really worried because I knew that it wasn't time yet for the birth. Needless to say, I was very concerned about my baby's health. My mom and dad raced me to the hospital. A short time later, I gave birth to my son, Ryan Michael. He was premature, jaundiced, and had fluid in his lungs. I was absolutely terrified.

In recovery, I looked up and saw Mary—in spirit—standing by my bedside. "Mary, what are you doing here?" I asked her, astonished.

"I told you I wanted to be there when you had your baby," she said. "He is so beautiful! He will be fine and strong."

I was so happy to see her! Then the nurse walked in and Mary disappeared.

A few months after Ryan was born, Mary appeared to me again. She was sitting on the edge of my bed. I was feeding Ryan at the time. Delighted to see her, I asked her why she was visiting. Mary told me that she was at peace, and that I should no longer worry about her. I was thrilled by Mary's message, so I called her mom, and she surprised me by sharing that Mary had also visited her the same night . . . to relay a similar message!

Since then, Ryan has grown into a strong, healthy man, just as Mary had promised. I hear her beautiful sweet voice at those times when I need reassurance the most. Our friendship has continued to prevail over time and space, and I have faith that, until I return to heaven myself, she'll always be there for me.

As a woman, you might find yourself asking, *Why do I have so much of the responsibility? I'm the one who conceives, I'm the one who carries the baby, I'm the one who gives birth, I'm the one who has to physically and emotionally heal after a miscarriage or birth, I'm the one who fixes up the nursery, takes care of the home, and—at the same time—I have some of the responsibility of bringing money into the household! Why is there so much on my shoulders?*

It's all true! Might it be said that shouldering all of these responsibilities provides you with a feeling of empowerment and achievement? You're a woman! You can juggle five hundred balls in the air—before breakfast! Celebrate your ability to multitask. Throughout history, women have proven that it is possible to encounter challenge—or adversity—and rise above it, continuing to follow their dreams and passions. Think of struggle as something that can *fuel* your forward movement rather than derail it. No matter what anyone else believes, the only thing that matters is what is in your own heart.

You are the architect of your life. In the final analysis, you won't be able to blame, or hold responsible, anyone else for the things you chose not to accomplish. Always follow your dreams, no matter how hard the struggle! If it is your destiny to become a parent, I believe you will be able to make that happen . . . although it may not be in the exact time frame or manner in which you envision.

Melissa's Story

I had tried to get pregnant for about a year and was getting very discouraged. I like to exercise, and during a run one day, I heard a voice very clearly inside my head say, "Don't worry, Mom, I'm coming!" I was a little startled, but I decided to answer the unexpected voice.

"Really?" I said. "Because it feels like it's taking forever!"

Then the voice responded, "I promise I'm coming soon, and I'm going to be a really good boy."

From that moment on, I started to relax a bit more and began to talk to him in my head whenever I got discouraged.

His answer always was, "Don't worry, Mom, I'm coming!"

A month later I was pregnant. From that moment on, I

routinely told my unborn baby how much I loved him and that I was so happy and grateful he was growing in my belly.

Throughout the pregnancy, he always responded in the sweetest voice, telling me that he was so happy to be mine as well. I felt like I had forged a very strong connection to him long before he was born.

The first night in the hospital, after his birth, he wasn't sleeping well so I put him in my arms and slept with him there the entire night. I quickly discovered that I could get him really relaxed if I just held him next to me. He is the sweetest little angel who loves being next to his mommy.

When an unborn baby chooses his birth mother, that is just the first step in the process. The baby does not have complete control over conception and pregnancy. He needs you, your partner, and in rare instances, your healthcare provider—as illustrated in Peggy's story at the end of this chapter—to make his return to the earthly plane a reality.

For example, an unborn baby might have his heart set on a particular birth mother, even if she has fertility challenges or lifestyle issues that could potentially derail the pregnancy. The unborn baby understands that if his chosen birth mother does not address these issues, then ultimately, his opportunity to return to the earthly plane—to that particular mother—might be denied him.

Think of conception and pregnancy as a bond of mutual trust between you and the baby. When you want to start a family, you trust that an unborn baby will choose you as a mother. Once that happens, the unborn baby trusts you to conceive and make the positive lifestyle choices that will result in a health pregnancy, labor, and delivery.

Therefore, once your baby has chosen you as his mother, as well as the approximate day and time of his birth, he then depends on you and your partner to do your part to conceive and maintain a healthy pregnancy. While it is true that the baby may decide to end the pregnancy through a miscarriage, that remains unlikely. Remember all of the positive statistics you just read about? So let's discuss what a woman can do, for her part, to conceive and maintain a pregnancy that is as healthy as possible.

The key to conceiving is to remain focused on your goal. You have an essential mission to accomplish. Think of yourself as an athlete. You are in training for an all-important contest that is certain to change your life . . . like the Olympics! Conceiving is better than any gold medal, but think of it in those terms. However, unlike the Olympic Games that are held every four years, you can get pregnant any time a soul is ready to be born. The most vital task at hand is to connect with sperm.

When I was trying to get pregnant, I'll wager I had more resolute determination than General George S. Patton when he was strategizing the D-Day invasion. I had my task at hand, and I knew that if I wasn't vigilant, my babies would never be born. It was up to me. And now, your time is at hand. It's up to you.

As a psychic channel in private practice, I've received a lot of valuable information for clients from their guardian angels and unborn babies about conception and pregnancy that I'm sharing below, along with advice from authorities including a respected OB/GYN, a female internist who has five children, a midwife, and a hypnotherapist. I hope you find it insightful and enlightening.

Conception and Pregnancy Tips—Round 1

I begin with advice my clients have received from their guardian angels and unborn babies in private channeling sessions conducted over the last twenty-two years.

Don't forget to smell the roses during this amazing time in your life. Spending sexual time with your sweetie when you are mutually interested in conceiving is a magical experience. You'll never have these moments back again. Plus, don't worry—about worrying! While your doctor may suggest that it is imperative to maintain a harmonious lifestyle while trying to conceive, that is sometimes easier in theory than in practice. If you're like me, you may experience a combination of stress, unhappiness, anger, nervous anticipation, frustration, fear, worry, and depression—before breakfast—because of trying to conceive. Do the very best you can. I admit that I do not have a medical degree, but I believe that if a serene state of mind was that imperative to the process, no one would ever conceive.

In the Middle Ages, women conceived and gave birth typically in what we would consider to be very unfavorable conditions. For instance, families bathed infrequently and in a single tub. For some inexplicable reason, the man of the house—who was arguably the dirtiest person in the family—would bathe first.

When he was finished, his wife would climb into the same grimy bathwater, and when she was through, it was time to bathe the babies and children. By that time, the water was so murky and foul that the expression was coined, "Don't throw the baby out with the bathwater."

In contrast, you probably have plenty of clean water to drink, cook with, and bathe in; a roof over your head; enough food to eat; prenatal vitamins; proper clothing; decent medical care; a significant other who wants you to be the mother of his children; and a uterus to make it all possible. The world is your oyster!

Have frequent sex. During a private channeling session, I once had a client inquire as to why she wasn't able to get pregnant. Her angels quickly responded by reminding her that she was only having sex twice a month! The process I have heard guardian angels recommend more than any other in my private channeling sessions is this: whatever day your period begins—even if you are only spotting a little—is Day One. Starting on Day Ten, have sex *every day* until your period starts again. It doesn't matter what position or what time of day. Did you know that sperm can remain alive inside of you for up to forty-eight hours after ejaculation?

Also, pay attention to Mr. Wonderful's fertility as well. Are you aware that, even if it's chilly outside, men can get very hot and sweaty under their testicles, just like we can get moist under our breasts? If the testicles are overheated, it reduces the sperm count and makes for sluggish swimmers. You can easily, quickly, and affordably do something about this! Get a small portable fan. Position it on a table in front of the couch, a chair, or the bed.

Ask your sweetheart to undress and then recline—maybe with some reading material—so that the fan can blow directly on his testicles for about twenty minutes. Make sure that the air blowing on your sweetheart's nether-regions is cool . . . *not* cold, so he's comfortable. After twenty minutes, turn off the fan and make love *immediately*, in any position. Although I am certainly not a physician, nor do I diagnose fertility problems, I have had several healthy clients over the years who have expressed frustration with their attempts to conceive. When I conducted a private channeling session for them, the fan advice was obtained from their guardian angels. By employing this simple technique, several of them were able to conceive a short time later!

After my miscarriage, I was plagued with sinus infections, sore throats, continual nasal drainage, colds, fatigue, and episodes of bronchitis. My sinus infections would always turn bacterial, and I'd be sick as a dog, which forced me to cancel a great number of private sessions that people had waited so long to have. I would make yet another appointment with my E.N.T. and he would prescribe another round of antibiotics. Although I believed that one of the underlying causes of my unstable health was my emotions, I was shocked to learn—from my guardian angels—that the real underlying cause was yeast toxicity! I didn't realize that someone could be toxic with yeast. When I reflected upon my eating habits, it became obvious. I was consuming a *lot* of yeast. Breads, pasta, salads with vinegar dressing, mushrooms, bananas, chips . . . and, to my greater dismay, I learned that refined sugar only added to the problem. Think of what happens when you dissolve one of those small packets of dry yeast in warm water and then add a small amount of sugar. A few years before, I had abandoned my healthy eating habits and had begun to consume a boatload of refined sugar, as well as juice and fruit. Plus, all the rounds of antibiotics I was taking added to the yeast toxicity.

I found an allergist in my area, Dr. Steven Hotze, the author of *Hormones, Health, and Happiness* and one of the foremost authorities on yeast, hormone, thyroid, and allergy disorders. He listened to me describe my symptoms and prescribed an oral, naturally compounded progesterone, and he also suggested some thorough testing be performed to allow him to make other evaluations. He discovered that my yeast count was through the roof! So I put off trying to get pregnant and began a three-month cleanse under his supervision. During the cleanse, I took the pharmaceutical Nystatin, prescribed by Dr. Hotze, to clean out the yeast that was already in my system and undermining my health, while at the same time eliminating all the yeast products from my eating habits. Shortly after that, I began to feel like a million bucks. In spite of the fact that I lived in Houston, arguably one of the sinus and allergy capitals of the world, I was rarely troubled by sinus or headaches after conducting the cleanse. Moreover, I believe that cleaning out my system from all of that yeast helped me conceive faster and enjoy healthier pregnancies, which was what I could do—for my part—to provide my babies the best physical environment possible in which their little bodies could grow. The major symptoms of yeast toxicity include: achy joints, gas, sinus congestion, constipation, nasal drainage, sore throats, headaches, fatigue, problems with weight loss, as well as a strong craving for the foods that are causing all of the problems! Does everyone have an issue with yeast? No, of course not. But if you've been suffering from these symptoms, or any other health-related issue, it wouldn't hurt to check it out *before* you attempt to conceive.

Conception and Pregnancy Tips—Round 2

Geoffrey Schnider, M.D., P.A., is a fellow of the American College of Obstetrics and Gynecology, a diplomate of the American Board of Obstetrics and Gynecology, and an active staff member of Woman's Hospital of Texas. Dr. Schnider states that he loves the science of obstetrics and taking care of women and delivering babies, combined with the surgery involved in gynecology. Because so many women are delaying pregnancy, as I had, I asked him to share his thoughts on the over-thirty-five obstetrical patients. I clearly remembered that before I conceived, he had tried to gently point out the challenges I might face as an older woman so I could be better informed. Dr. Schnider told me that in his practice he "has no problem at all once a woman is informed of the risks and the initial hurdle of ensuring normal genetic testing is overcome, and the patient is in reasonable health, the older mother's pregnancy may proceed in much the same way as any other."

As someone who has consistently been voted one of Houston's best doctors, I asked Dr. Schnider to present some of the advice that he gives patients in regard to conception and pregnancy.

When a woman is planning to conceive, she needs to live as clean a life as possible—as if she was already pregnant. Dr. Schnider reminds patients that once they have passed ovulation, they should—to be on the safe side—assume that they're pregnant. He points out that a woman has already been pregnant for two weeks before she misses a period.

"At the same time," he says, "patients tend nowadays to become very worked up if they haven't gotten pregnant after a couple of tries. They need to give it a little time, and not make a lab experiment out of what should be a natural process."

Weeks before conception, avoid medications that can affect the pregnancy. In general, avoid as much medication as possible, and take only what is necessary. Your physician should provide you with a list of medications that are not advised, as well as those that are safe to ingest before and during pregnancy. For example, certain medications are absolutely not recommended because they are known to cause birth defects. Most medications are cleared from the body very quickly, while others remain stored in a woman's fat tissue for weeks, or longer. If a patient has any doubts, she needs to check with her physician *before* she takes a medication.

Avoid extreme heat, such as saunas, steam baths, hot tubs, and hot baths while trying to conceive or if already pregnant, as it can raise the core body temperature to levels that are unsafe and harmful to the baby.

Conception and Pregnancy Tips—Round 3

When I was ready to conceive again about six months after my miscarriage, I was fortunate to have dinner with a girlfriend who I consider to be Super Woman. Elisa Medhus is an internist, the mother of five, and the author of three award-winning books on parenting, including *Raising Children Who Think for Themselves.* I mentioned my situation to her, and she began to share some fertility advice that I had never heard before.

Elisa began by disclosing that her sister-in-law had suffered from a series of miscarriages, and that once she had taken Elisa's advice—she had proceeded to give birth to three healthy children! Although all women are different, and it's true that destiny plays a huge role in how and when we conceive and give birth, it's important to remember that you have to do your part to make all of your baby dreams possible. If you have had a history of early miscarriages or have had trouble conceiving in the first place, Dr. Elisa offers a number of recommendations that are relatively safe and often highly effective. Please note that some of her advice involves pharmaceutical agents, so you'll have to get your own doctor's approval—and prescriptions—before considering any of Dr. Elisa's suggestions:

Take one 81mg baby aspirin daily from the day you begin trying to conceive all the way through your third month of pregnancy. Some women make proteins called "autoantibodies" against naturally occurring molecules in the body. One such molecule is called cardiolipin, a building block for the membranes in our cells' mitochondria.

Mitochondria are small power factories inside our cells. That said, when we attack cardiolipin with anticardiolipin antibodies, we're essentially attacking the embryo's cells. This often results in a miscarriage, sometimes before a woman even knows she's pregnant. In fact, these miscarriages often fly under the radar screen as a heavy menstrual period. Baby aspirin minimizes inflammation, which includes autoimmune reactions.

Progesterone: It is vital for you to have enough progesterone in your system.Progesterone is one of the female hormones necessary for implantation of the fertilized egg to occur in the uterine wall and to maintain that implantation throughout the pregnancy. For women with a history of multiple miscarriages, some physicians recommend progesterone supplementation every day for the first trimester, which is the first three months of your pregnancy.

Treating bacterial vaginitis: Many women are completely unaware that they have a chronic vaginal infection known as gardnerella vaginitis, also known as bacterial vaginitis. Not an STD, it can persist in the vagina for years. It is known to possibly cause pelvic inflammatory disease, endometritis, amniotic fluid infection, preterm delivery, preterm labor, premature rupture of the membranes, and miscarriage. Two of the most effective treatments for bacterial vaginitis include an oral medication called Flagyl (metronidazole), and the intravaginal antibiotic clindamycin ovules. As long as the mother has finished her dosage of either of these two medications at least seven days before conceiving, the baby should be fine.

Prenatal vitamins that contain folic acid and DHA: During pregnancy, the baby takes what nutrients it needs from you, often leaving your body depleted of important substrates. While a nutritious diet is vital, prenatal vitamins ensure that the gaps are filled and provide you with the ever-important folic acid. Folic acid can reduce certain birth defects of the brain and spinal cord by more than 70 percent. Folic acid may also help lower your chances of getting heart disease, some types of cancer, and may also help protect you from having a stroke. DHA is an omega-3 fatty acid that helps your baby's developing brain. DHA, a phospholipid building block of nerve membranes, comprises around 80 percent of the weight of the brain. Americans tend to be severely deficient in omega-3s, and many in the medical community believe the rise in mental health disorders like ADHD and bipolar disease are caused in part by this deficit. Prenatal vitamins always contain multivitamins and folic acid. Dr. Elisa highly recommends that women take prenatal vitamins during pregnancy, and if possible, for one year prior to getting pregnant.

Important tests to conduct once pregnant: complete blood count, urine analysis, thyroid functions, chemistry profile, blood type with Rh factor and antibodies, HIV, syphilis, hepatitis B immunity, and rubella antibodies.

Time to begin considering fertility treatments: Dr. Elisa would begin the evaluation process if the patient was under thirty and had suffered a second miscarriage, or after the first miscarriage if the woman is over thirty. She would wait at least two years to start fertility treatments, depending on the individual couple, including age, financial status, and levels of patience. The type of treatment would depend on whether the primary problem stemmed from difficulties with conception or miscarriages. Before considering actually fertility treatment, these all have to be evaluated in depth.

Conception and Pregnancy Tips—Round 4

Melanie Dossey, a certified nurse midwife, graduate of the renowned Baylor College of Medicine Midwifery, and owner of the Nativiti Women's Health & Birth Center, has been helping women conceive and give birth for over twenty years. Her busy practice has increasingly represented more mature mothers, reflecting one of the fastest growing segments of the pregnancy market. "I would like the medical community to redo some of the research that scares woman away from having babies later in life. They should not be afraid! I recently had a forty-eight-year-old patient give birth to a healthy baby."

Melanie advises her patients, "I want everything that passes through your lips to be as healthy as possible. That is the portal to make nutrition for the human you are growing in your body, so think about food as part of the gasoline that you're putting into your system. Don't be around smokers, don't be around marijuana, because airborne substances can absorb into the fat of your body and remain there for possibly up to six months."

For her patients interested in holistic health, nutrition, and homeopathy, she recommends the book, *Wise Woman Herbal*, written by Susan Weed. The book shares information about herbal and homeopathic remedies to help regulate menstrual cycles, stem bleeding during pregnancy, and a host of other female health concerns and interests.

Please note: Some of her advice involves mineral and vitamin supplements, so you'll have to get your own doctor's (or midwife's) approval before following any of these suggestions:

B6 is known as the "stress vitamin." Taken with Benadryl 25mg, it can help alleviate some symptoms related to morning sickness. One of my clients recently found a nutritional source online: http://www.karenhurd.com/ morningsickness.html (Karen Hurd, a nutritionist, and the author of the website, doesn't agree with my B6 philosophies, but I've found it to be effective.) My client tried the Hurd legume remedy for her morning sickness, and she said black beans cured her nausea in three days.

Skip dairy products and coffee in early pregnancy because they can cause morning sickness; many women are lactose intolerant, so often a calcium supplement works best—in addition to a one-a-day prenatal multivitamin. Besides helping a pregnant woman feed her own bones and those of her baby's, calcium supplements can help eliminate painful leg cramps that often occur at 24–26 weeks of pregnancy.

Do not take calcium and iron at the same time. Together, they will cause constipation. Calcium and iron taken together will clash, reducing their absorption and canceling out their health benefits, while drinking milk with an iron supplement will cause the same effect.

To help conceive, use progesterone cream, a quarter teaspoon twice a day from the time you are trying to conceive through your third month of pregnancy. Simply rub it into your skin.

Eliminate tobacco and alcohol before trying to conceive

Wait at least six months to conceive after recreational drug use (including exposure to marijuana) because remnants of those chemicals can remain in your fat cells long-term.

Conception and Pregnancy Tips—Round 5

After you've conceived—or even *before* conception—consider scheduling some private sessions with a reputable hypnotherapist. It is possible that you could minimize discomfort during labor and shorten your delivery time though hypnotic suggestion. In spite of the fact that I planned to get an epidural, I was really scared about my first labor and delivery and simply couldn't imagine how a big baby was going to pass through such a little area. So I decided to try something that had helped in other areas of my life—I made an appointment with Houston hypnotherapist Carolyn H. Grace.

I told Carolyn that my goal was to shorten my labor and delivery while allowing it to be as comfortable as possible. I wanted to enjoy every moment of that miraculous experience. I left the hypnotherapy sessions feeling tremendously relaxed and centered.

Does hypnosis really work, you ask? All I can tell you is that when I was forty-four years old, my first labor lasted a little over five hours, from the moment I felt the first little twinge at home to the time when my eight-pound, three-ounce son, Flynn, popped out of my body at the hospital. I felt such peace the moment I gave birth to my son that I surprised Dr. Schnider by excitedly telling him that I would be back the following year to give birth to my daughter—and that I couldn't wait. If memory serves, he said something to the effect of, "I've never had a patient give birth, and while I'm still stitching her, tell me that she's looking forward to repeating the process!"

Hypnotherapist Carolyn Grace, who so dramatically helped me relax and enjoy both of my births, shares her experiences and beliefs about what may be accomplished with the use of hypnosis for conception, pregnancy, and childbirth in the information below.

Hypnosis aids in:

The process of conception by overcoming anxiety, stress, dread, or fear of pregnancy or childbirth

Helps the mother communicate with her baby in utero and during birthing

Creates a general state of relaxation and calmness, which benefits the health and well-being of both mother and fetus during pregnancy

Helps the mother overcome fear of needles and other medical procedures associated with pregnancy and/or childbirth

Eliminates or reduces morning sickness or nausea

Decreases hypertension associated with pregnancy

Reduces headaches, insomnia, and back pain

Can provide a less strenuous labor and birth process by minimizing anxiety and fear, thus reducing pain and resulting in a more positive experience both mentally and physically

Can potentially shorten labor because you learn to focus and thus become more relaxed

Can decrease the need for medications and their associated risks for mother and/or baby

Decreases the need for surgical intervention, forceps, or Cesarean section

Decreases chances of an episiotomy because in a relaxed state, the perineum—the area surrounding the vagina and anus—becomes more elastic

Promotes a more rapid recovery process following childbirth; the mother is less mentally and physically exhausted/stressed

Much less stress on baby; babies have been shown to cry less, sleep better, and feed better. They are generally calmer

Decreases chances of postnatal and/or postpartum depression

The following true-life story illustrates how Peggy—emotionally desolate after a series of miscarriages and a failed fertility treatment—mustered the strength, courage, and resolve to try again . . . inspired by the spirit of her unborn daughter.

Peggy's Story

A green tennis ball sailed over the net, whisking past the opposing player.

"Whew!" Coach Peter whistled through his teeth. "Did you eat your spinach today, Caitlin?"

"No . . ." Caitlin smiled, a blush rising to her cheeks.

My eyes sparkled with a mother's pride. Was that *my* little girl pounding that ball? It was hard to believe there was a time when Catie wasn't a part of our lives, our hopes, or our future. A breeze lifted my bangs. I stared ahead. Catie and her teammates blurred . . . their voices faded and I was transported to a time before Caitlin . . . a time when her presence existed only in my dreams, my thoughts, and my intuition.

My husband, Tommy, and I were at home in our den consumed with nervous anticipation when the phone rang. Tommy answered. Dr. Lila suggested my husband hug me. The first in vitro procedure had failed. I wasn't pregnant. After squeezing me tight, Tommy turned to leave. After three miscarriages prior to this in vitro attempt, my husband wore a protective emotional armor that nothing could penetrate. A huge lump rose in my throat. My eyes welled, but no tears came; strangely, neither did the deep pain that I was expecting.

I felt despair so penetrating that only God could understand my presence of mind in that terrible time. I yearned to be a mother, and I didn't know what to do. I considered the options available to us. We could adopt, or we could try using donor eggs. Or we could try in vitro again.

At that moment, an inner knowing suddenly took hold and began to soothe me. Was the inner voice coming from my unborn baby, I wondered? Steeling myself, I acknowledged that I had to persevere or we would never achieve our dream of having a child. The soothing knowingness inside my head helped me decide on the right course of action for my husband and me. I decided to forego using donor eggs or adoption. In spite of all of the unsolicited advice and opinions from other people, and the depressing statistics of success on this costly procedure, I just *knew* we had to try a second course of in vitro.

The next few weeks felt blurred, like traveling through a wind tunnel at a speed faster than light. Needles, ultrasounds, and the doctor visits melted together. To my surprise, everything went much smoother than the first time . . . even when my specialist took a vacation during the implantation process. All the while, there was a constant stream of comforting emotional knowingness that provided me support and encouragement.

Finally, blood was drawn to determine whether I was pregnant. An unwavering calm enveloped me as I left the lab to drive back to work. It was an inner peace that I had never experienced before. No stomach flutters. No rapid heartbeat. All of the negative symptoms that were common for me during the first in vitro procedure were amazingly absent. This state of serenity was completely unknown to me—a woman who family and friends often referred to as the Type A personality poster child.

I waited until twelve o'clock to make the call to the doctor's office. "Are my results in?" I questioned, my voice barely a whisper. The nurse asked me to hold while she located the doctor. I bit my lip and waited.

"How are you feeling?" asked Dr. Lila, the moment she came to the phone. Her voice had a steady, matter-of-fact tone.

"Fine," I responded curtly. My heart began to race. My breathing quickened. "Just tell me!"

"Well . . . how would you like to be a mom?"

My breath caught in my chest. Did I hear correctly?

"Because you're going to be one!" the doctor announced. "Congratulations!"

I managed to say thank you before hanging up. In a single moment, my life had changed forever! Tears ran down my cheeks. I closed my eyes, savoring the joy. Our dream had come true! There was a living, breathing miracle inside of me.

A few months later, I had a sonogram. My heart leaped when I saw the tiny face on the screen. A smile was clearly visible, and the baby seemed to be staring back at me. "Here I am, Mom!" I actually heard inside my head. "I'll see you soon!"

The final months of the pregnancy were filled with anxiousness, anticipation, and longing. Fear would sometimes reign as well. We decided not to buy a crib until I was eight months along. But then . . . the day came.

With one last push, I closed my eyes and suddenly saw my deceased mother, Dorothy. Mom smiled and waved. And then, Caitlin Elizabeth was in my arms. My baby was really here!

"Peg," my husband murmured softly. "She looks just like your mom."

I smiled down at the newest member of our family.

Suddenly, I was jarred back to the present. "Mom! *Mom*! How did I do?" Catie's big brown eyes stared back at me. Her forehead was beaded with sweat as she waved goodbye to her teammates.

"What?" I answer a bit sheepishly. "Oh . . . great!" The fog had broken and I was back in the moment. As I listened to my daughter talk excitedly about her tennis lesson, I glanced around at the other families. Some of the parents were laughing, some scolding, some were talking quietly with their children. I wondered if they realized the "miracles" in their midst?

The road was hard for my husband and me to have our beautiful child. We experienced the magic first hand when the intuitive *knowing* foretold the possibility of an incredible gift that turned into a reality.

Pulling out of the parking lot, I glanced at the ponytailed little girl sitting next to me. I thanked God for her existence and for giving me the determination, strength, and courage years before to follow my heart . . . and fulfill our destiny.

I wish you the greatest joy and peace as you embark on the most profound spiritual adventure of all—parenthood! May the days to come be filled with the angelic sound of your child's laughter, and your own wonderment of the miracle that you helped create.

ABOUT THE AUTHOR

Kim O'Neill, recently voted Houston's top psychic by *Houston Press Magazine*, is the author of *How to Talk with Your Angels* and *Discover Your Spiritual Destiny* (both by Harper-Collins Books), and the self-published *The Calling, Journey of a Psychic*.

For more than twenty-two years, she has conducted private channeling sessions for an international list of clients that include physicians, judges, attorneys, professionals in the entertainment industry, politicians, college professors, foreign dignitaries, religious leaders, fellow psychics, private investigators, police departments, FBI agents, Secret Service agents, authors, artists, corporate executives, radio DJs, newspaper and television reporters, as well as hosts of television talk shows.

Kim has established international motivational seminars and workshops designed to help people transform their lives and develop greater spiritual awareness. She also writes *Connecting You*

With Spirit, a monthly EMagazine, as well as a monthly advice column called *Ask Kim* for the *Indigo Sun Magazine*. Kim has channeled for radio and television talk show audiences, providing accurate and specific psychic information covering a wide range of topics. She lives in Houston, Texas, with her husband and their two children.

Author's Note

I conduct private sessions by telephone, host teleseminars, and present in-person workshops across the United States and Canada. I would love to be of service to you! I can be reached through my office: 281-651-1599; or on my website: www.kimoneill psychic.com.

If you have a baby story of your own, please e-mail me. I might include it in my next book!